GIFT OF TIME

GIFT OF TIME

Rory MacLean
with Joan and Katrin MacLean

Constable • London

Constable & Robinson Ltd
3 The Lanchesters
162 Fulham Palace Road
London W6 9ER
www.constablerobinson.com

First published in the UK by Constable,
an imprint of Constable & Robinson Ltd., 2011

A copy of the British Library Cataloguing in
Publication data is available from the British Library

ISBN 978-1-84901-857-9

Typeset by TW Typesetting, Plymouth, Devon

Printed and bound in the UK

1 3 5 7 9 10 8 6 4 2

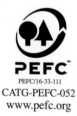

PEFC

PEFC/16-33-111
CATG-PEFC-052
www.pefc.org

And did you get what
you wanted from this life, even so?
I did.
And what did you want?
To call myself beloved, to feel myself
beloved on the earth.

Late Fragment, Raymond Carver

Preface

I don't think of you every day now. I no longer expect to wake at night and see you smiling at me from the end of the bed. I don't glimpse your face in a crowd or repeat your phone number over and over in my head like the coda from one of your scratched, Broadway musical LPs. It has been seven years since I held your hand, since you took your last breath and I opened the bedroom window to let your soul fly free. I never thought it would happen.

Do you remember our plan to stay in touch? We never speculated which one of us would be the first to go. It was always going to be you of course, fatal accident or natural disaster notwithstanding. The vast majority of parents die before their children. But whoever went first, we agreed to try to send the survivor a sign, a kind of cosmic postcard reporting, 'Tremendously busy here, craic good, did you return the books to the library?' We would show that life wasn't simply a biological phenomena, that death was a kind of evolution, that love endured beyond the grave.

In the days immediately after your death I believed you were still near. I felt your presence in the next room, somewhere above your golden armchair. Then I sensed you standing behind me, here in my study. At any moment I expected to catch your reflection in my computer's screen. I made two cups of blackcurrant tea in faith as much as out of habit. I waited for you to tap me on the shoulder and remind me that 'credulity' is spelt with one 't'. I felt your warmth on my back, on my neck, against my ear.

But like a dying fire, the warmth faded away. I could no longer deny that you had been zipped into a black body bag and carried away, the stretcher's metal frame gouging a finger's length from the wallpaper. I came to see our pact for what it was, an illusion conjured up to protect soft hearts from hard truth. I could no longer believe that you were off on an adventure, that your spirit lived on, that we would meet again one day. There would be no postcard from the hereafter; there is no other place apart from this lone, high-skied paradise. With that understanding I ceased to be the whimsical, gentle child you had raised. Your love had nurtured me in a way that allowed me to believe in my own uniqueness. After you had gone, I became ordinary. I was no longer invincible. I stumbled and fell. On the platform at Victoria station I wept.

Since then you've come to me only in wishes. I wish that you'd left us your granola recipe and that I'd known sooner about your love for Formula One racing. I wish that you could have seen me this morning winding the battered travel clock that you gave to me on the day I moved away from home, winding and winding it so that its brass heartbeat might never stop. I wish you'd been beside me in the shadows last night, watching Katrin gaze at another world in that joyful photograph of us, light and laughing in your kitchen one year before the diagnosis. I wish you could meet your five-year-old grandson Finn, bent over your old Smith-Corona, typing his first book (*The Sea and the View* – God knows where he got that from) on three sheets of A4 stapled together. I want you to ring the doorbell right now, refuse an offer of tea so as not to disturb my writing and invite us to the Cottage for Sunday dinner.

I read somewhere that we don't work through grief but that it works through us, that it is a process. In the first years I lost patience, humour and joy. Time has helped me through the process, as have Katrin, family and friends; as does Finn. Day by day, through him, I rediscover joy (as well as an ability to design eccentric bubble-blowing machines). Our hours together are as precious as any love that anticipates death, for its unwanted shadow has grafted itself to me.

Until a few months ago I still found it hard to open these diaries. Now all our thoughts are interwoven, your handwritten pages and Post-its with our bubble-jet typescripts. The book is a way of bringing all of us together again. But writing is also part of who I am, just as reading was part of who you were. I perceive the world by rendering it into words. I distil experience, portraying the world as I perhaps wish it could be (you remember as a child I made a card-and-crayon world atlas in which imaginary lands and stories were interleaved with the countries I knew). This longing for a more intense reality reaches back to those first happy years of childhood, to a lost world, which I have often tried to recreate in my writing.

However exclusive every grief may be, there are still many aspects of it that are shared. In your quiet and gallant way you showed us how self-discipline and love can delay the end. By strength of will you ordered your lungs to keep breathing and your heart to keep beating. You let us be a part of your struggle and dying and that was a privilege, a gift. Now in a time of changing sensibilities our experience may help others, and their families, to face death at home with dignity, to have *una bella morte* – a good death, as the Italians say – surrounded by family and friends, in peace.

Last night in a dream Katrin gave me a child's plastic telescope. 'Look through it and you may see your Mum,' she told me. Slowly, with a mixture of excitement and trepidation, I lifted the spy-glass to my eye.

December

Thursday 30th

Rory: Crisp winter's day. Hard frost. High blue sky. Ice underfoot. This morning Mum comes home. I pick her up from the hospital. Barbara, the ward sister, wheels her out to the car. As I lower her into the passenger seat she holds onto my neck, as light as a pillowcase of bones. Barbara says twice, 'Your family want you to go home with them.'

None of the other patients had visitors over Christmas. In the ward linger a dozen abandoned souls: Mary, a seventy-five-year-old ballroom dancer who lost both a leg and a husband last month ('It was a good life until Will died'); diabetic Jerry who won't eat ('Just one piece of toast,' entreats a nurse. 'I'll give you jam.'); Mrs Windsor who has caught the ward cough ('Any jobs for me?' she rasps five times a day, pleading to be useful, unable to lift herself out of bed. 'Can I arrange the flowers again?'). Two rings of beds in which tired, cadaverous bodies snore, wee and hawk into plastic beakers marked 'Sputum'. I smell antiseptic and fear. I hear the last rites being read behind a cheerful NHS curtain. Day and night a frail widower calls out for his wife. 'Liz . . . Liz . . . Ma . . .' Another geriatric stares at me, his eyes not moving, not even focusing. The English have been notoriously poor at handling death, hiding away feelings and relatives at one of life's most emotional moments, condemning themselves to years of inhibition and blocked grief. I'm not leaving Mum here to die alone. She is the only patient in the ward with her own teeth.

On the drive back to our village I put my hand on her leg. It feels bone thin. Only last month we walked together around the churchyard, her hand in the crook of my arm. She squeezes my hand. 'At least we have this gift of time together,' she says.

Yesterday I bought her a new diary. I carried from her cottage a cardboard box of family photographs. On the chest in the spare room I set her favourite portrait of my father, on the bridge of a corvette gazing out to sea. In a corner I positioned her golden armchair, a towel on its seat. On the bedside table I stacked her unopened Christmas cards. Half-a-dozen house plants crowded the window sill. I stowed our own things in the attic, to be put back at a later date. In the evening I practised piggy-backing Katrin up and down the stairs. Now she awaits us at the front door.

'I feel so happy to be home,' Mum tells her as I carry her into her new home. Her last home.

Joan: *That* was a wholly unexpected Christmas location. On Friday I was downstairs at the Cottage when my left leg suddenly seized up. Thankfully, Rita the occupational therapist happened to arrive with various walking sticks, but it was clear that this time I couldn't get upstairs, even with her help. An ambulance with two hearty helpers arrived twenty minutes later.

I felt sad to leave the tree and presents but the hospital made a real effort to create a festive atmosphere with streamers of tinsel and coloured decorations. The nursing staff were caring and helpful with a warmth and natural inclination to care and cosset: children, the sick, anything in distress. But the Yeatman is a hospital like any other with inevitable noise and, most disturbing at night, the snoring and coughing. Any illusion that women are delicate, fragile creatures was burst in shattering reverberations.

On 25th we sat around small tables with crackers, and a huge traditional Christmas dinner appeared, though the turkey was orthopaedic without appendages. The senior surgeon carved the bird and a few carol singers braved the dreadful storm. To my delight M suddenly walked in – wonderful and completely unexpected to see her as she was supposed to be with her fiancé, Mike. She looked lovely and brought a huge bunch of my favourite roses. We had such a dear chat about her happiness with Mike's – soon to be her – family.

Reading David Guterson's *East of the Mountains*: a masculine book written in a conversational style – story is of a plan to commit a staged suicide to avoid the long-drawn-out effects of cancer upon the body.

'I didn't want to burden my family . . . didn't want to make them miserable.'

'It isn't a burden,' said Bea. 'Think what they will learn from it.'

Katrin: How typical of Joan not to want us to change our Christmas plans, to wait until we had already left for my parents' before keeling over at the Cottage. However anxious we were to get back to her, at least we didn't have to worry about her being alone, or hurt, or frightened. This last month of uncertainty – of waiting for another call from Age Concern to tell us she's pressed her panic button – has been such a strain.

Dorset Social Services are going to send health workers starting next week, but until then I am again helping her to wash. While she was at the Cottage she could – with my help and some basic equipment – get into and out of the bath. Today even undressing is a struggle. It's frightening how much weaker she is only a few weeks later, but she is practical and unfussed by this turn of events. At least here we can really look after her. Her pale skin is flecked with minute age spots and gleams in the light. As I sponge her down I am moved by her vulnerability, by her petite feminine form, by her once beautiful, still slender body.

Friday 31st

Rory: Cold night. Crystal icing on the dry-stone walls. The low sun tightens a rosy collar around the horizon, picking out every black tree and frozen hedge on Knighton Hill. Katrin and I slept little, listening to her cough, waiting for her to ring the hand bell. I wheeled the trapdoor commode over the toilet bowl at midnight, three o'clock and six. 'I don't think we'll be overly concerned about modesty, darling,' she wheezed, as I helped her pull down her trousers. The morphine hardly suppresses the cough but it does constipate her. In yesterday's rush, collecting eleven prescriptions from the hospital pharmacy, I didn't notice that they'd forgotten the laxative. I should have checked.

Four weeks ago, during her regular check-up at Dorchester, her chest X-ray appeared to be clear. There was no sign of a recurrent tumour. Our concern was with her niggling cough.

'I want it to go away,' Mum told the oncologist.

Dr Marsden felt her lymph glands. They were hard and enlarged. He replied, 'I don't think it will.'

One week later, on Friday 17th, Mum could hardly walk into his office.

'How are you today, Mrs MacLean?' he asked her.

'I think we're getting there,' she smiled, ever optimistic.

Ten days ago, alone at the Cottage, she stood up from her reading chair and fell down. She hit her head and then her panic button. Katrin bathed the blood off her silver hair. Mum insisted that we not change our plans, and spend Christmas with Katrin's parents in Kent.

For breakfast she swallows grapes, steroids and a home-brewed laxative of wheatgerm and flax. My sister Marlie calls to find how she's settling in. Afterwards Katrin walks Mum around the landing.

'Left right left right.'

At the hospital, Barbara taught her to talk to her limbs.

'Come on, left leg.' Her left leg doesn't respond. She falls back in her chair, winded. 'We take so many things for granted,' she says and cries.

Katrin and I hold her hands. Her slippers no longer fit her swollen feet. I lay my forehead against her warm skull and say, 'I'm sorry, Mum.'

'Me too.'

Katrin roasts a chicken for our new year's supper. We eat it on our laps in her room. Later there are stars and fireworks above the village. Church bells peal down the length of the Blackmore Vale, keeping Mum awake.

Katrin: A portrait of her. A clean eraser, a pale tinted sheet of Ingres paper, a broad finger of charcoal, a fistful of chalk pastels – flesh tones, greys and whites; these are my materials. The rubber describes soft lines on a page already blackened with the charcoal, picking out the palest greys of her hairline and defining the long cheeks and oval face. I work away the darkness, highlighting contours and structure – eye sockets, cheekbones, chin – by subtraction and negation. I add in where I have taken away, sculpting volume with coloured chalks, letting familiar features emerge as age and illness slip away.

Now my fingertips move light chalk tones across her temples, gently gathering her hair away from a low forehead to its habitual place, pinned behind her head. I smooth a translucent layer of pigment like a pale eye-shadow over the wide plains of her downcast eyelids. I model the bridge and slope of a fine nose to its tip. I flesh out her cheeks, smooth and supple in spite of her years. Then with a graphite pencil I carve the blunt lines of her expression, adding contrast and etching detail – a fine mesh of lines around her delicate eyes, their endearing down-ward tilt, the creases to east and west of her nose, which connect with the smiling corners of her lips. Finally, a ghostly thumbprint locates her long, flat earlobes – always adorned – which lie at almost the same latitude as a small mobile mouth. Small touches of colours – eyes, mouth, hair, teeth – emphasize her pallor.

January

Saturday 1st

Rory: Cough changes in the night. Snuffles at dawn. She spits grey phlegm. A virus caught in the ward? I fall back in bed and wake Katrin from a dream of cooking a miracle cure stir-fry. Her kitchen floor is knee-deep in trimmings of garlic and ginger.

The weather changes, too. I walk Mum around the landing then vanish with Tess the dog into the morning mist. It's my first time out of the house in two days. The sound of my footsteps is muffled by the damp air. I see no lights in any window. The other villagers are either dead or watching *Mary Poppins*.

At twelve an ambulance takes her to Dorchester for scans. I follow in the car. She looks so frail, like an injured bird in a blanket. But she's not in pain, thank God. In the oncology waiting room a nurse strokes the forehead of a groaning, aching patient. He looks like an estate agent. A *dying* estate agent. 'Thumbs up, eh?' she whispers to him. She doesn't wish us a happy new year. There is a run in her tights.

In the afternoon the CancerCare nurse, Carole, stops by the house, bringing support and an application for attendance allowance. I need to complete a DS1500 Report. The form begins, 'Sadly, some people suffer from a terminal illness.' I'm reminded of Kafka's truism. The point of life, he said, is that it stops.

Carole teaches me how to lift Mum out of a chair. I must ease my left fist under her left arm, my right hand under her right arm, then hoist and shuffle sideways, dancing towards the bed or the loo. Unfortunately, the fingers of her left hand are locking today. If Katrin is with us she can ease them free from the chair's arm. If not, I have to lean Mum against my hip and loosen their grip. Sometimes when lifting her up in bed, her hips and legs lock, leaving her as rigid as a shop mannequin.

At the front door Carole says to me, 'Your mother is not the sort of woman to turn her face to the wall and give up. The courage of people never ceases to astound me.'

I sprint to the shop to buy a bottle of wine to bolster mine.

Evening brings rain and gale-force winds. I sit with Mum, reading. Downstairs Katrin paints the shower room. That night she slips into a dream. She and Mum are lying in long grass, gazing up into a blue summer sky, when a small bird flies into view.

'Look Joan, a goldfinch.'

It alights in a hedgerow and they steal forward to catch a better glimpse of it. Before their eyes the bird turns into a little angel, glittering in the branches.

'An angel! An angel!'

But as they draw nearer, the apparition transforms itself into a black cat, snarling, ears back, teeth exposed, ready to attack. Katrin cries herself awake and out of the nightmare, her skin crawling as if she'd seen a ghost.

I sleep on, thinking I can cope.

Joan: This morning to Dorchester by ambulance for chest and brain scan. Very pleasant technicians. R managed to recall the ambulance team early so I was not hanging around. On the way back to the village came news of an accident at Grimstone – the route R was driving in the

Escort, so I felt a flood of relief to see him safely home. K brought more of my treasures from the Cottage. The green bedroom is now very comfortable. Calls from dear A and M, their voices so welcome. Rowntree's Fruit Pastilles prove soothing for my throat.

Sunday 2nd

Rory: Hung over. And *I've* caught the ward cough.

At nine, the first home-care assistant tumbles into the house, wafting stale cigarette smoke. 'I think we're getting there,' Mum tells her too, in good spirits at the start of her journey. Her eyes are surprisingly bright. She is calm and clear. 'With any luck we'll stave off this bug.'

Every two hours she spends twenty minutes on the toilet with the tap running. A wooden whistle waits on the window sill for her to alert us when she's finished. Her urine is the colour of rust. We establish a routine to help us get by, amazed how quickly it exhausts us, then traps us.

Katrin and I risk leaving her alone to dash through the rain and collect her Christmas tree, carrying it home fully decorated, leaving a glittering tinsel trail along the High Street. I rig a string of twinkling white fairy lights and clusters of midnight blue baubles above her armchair. Katrin plays a selection of carols. We open the presents around her: books, woolly tights and Wellington boots, chosen three weeks ago when Mum could still walk unaided. We laugh at the absurdity of the gift.

In a quiet moment she tells me, 'When you take down the tree, you children should divide the decorations. Next Christmas I can borrow back what I need.'

Monday 3rd

Rory: 'I'm feeling very sparky this morning. Perhaps we should drink champagne every night?'

Today Mum can open and close her left hand. She stands without support as Katrin washes her. She walks with head down and arms taut, pushing the Zimmer frame back and forth in two-inch steps between her bedroom, the bathroom, our bedroom and my study, the extent of her new world. I'm amazed that her condition can fluctuate so dramatically and the improvement enables me to get back to work. I perch at my desk writing a radio programme about adventure travel, about zorbing and white water rafting, as she shuffles through the room talking to her legs. There's an illusion of spring in the air.

Katrin makes a goat's cheese salad with raspberry vinegar dressing for lunch. Chicken on a bed of leeks for supper. The sour taste that Mum has had in her mouth for the last two weeks has gone. I ask her if she wants to watch television in her room. She shakes her head. 'I don't want to know about the outside. I'm very content here.' I pick her another selection of books.

Katrin christens our new shower room, cobbled together from family and friends' donations: glass cubicle from Putney, ceramic basin from Kent, tiles from Gloucestershire. Tess the retriever lies on the floor howling at her, wanting to be in the water.

I call Marlie in London and my brother Andrew in Toronto to update them. Marlie wants Mum to live with her in London. But Mum does not want her illness to intrude on the new life she is building.

'If I'd spoken to you two days ago, I'd have been less optimistic,' I say.

'But you know we're on a sliding scale,' Andrew tells me. 'There's only so much that you can cope with.'

Andrew wants me to put Mum into a home for the sake of *our* health.

Joan: Reading Diane Ackerman's *A Natural History of the Senses*: 'The peace of that moment crested over me like a breaking wave and saturated my senses.' R writing the new radio series with fierce concentration. Good interview with Julian Barnes. Each programme takes three days of writing, one day to record and airs in twenty-eight minutes.

Tuesday 4th

Rory: Dull day. The landscape is without contrast, as if its painter had mixed grey into all the colours on his palette. Katrin returns to work at Fired Earth so we're alone in the house. Mum settles down to proof-read the manuscript of my Florida book (with its seat lowered, the commode doubles as a chair-side desk). She has proofed every one of my books. Our editorial session is interrupted by visits from Rita the occupational therapist, Florence the district nurse and Frieda the physiotherapist. Social services ring twice. CancerCare Carole arranges to come by on Thursday. I forget to book an ambulance to take us to Dorchester on Friday for the results of the scan.

During our pre-lunch, inter-bedroom amble I measure how high Mum can lift her feet. Eight inches on the right. Three inches on the left. 'You could probably manage the stairs,' I suggest.

'I can't spare the energy to go downstairs,' she replies, shaking her head. 'When I find energy, I conserve it. That's what I'm doing now. Conserving.'

All her courage is being used up fighting the disease. She hasn't any left to confront the stairs.

In the evening, Marlie confirms that she can visit from London for the weekend. She's anxious about the scan results. She also wants to share her wedding plans.

Wednesday 5th

Joan: With the help of the humidifier, a sleeping pill and Oramorph, I slept right through the night – unbelievably refreshing! Naturally, awoke with chest congestion but walks have the nether regions working again. Began opening the Christmas cards and made a list of friends to call – I hope they'll forgive me for not sending letters this year. Also balanced my bank account. Luckily, enough money there for the Cottage rent.

The district nurse (a.k.a. Florence Nightingale) here again to write up her notes and chat rather woollily about acceptance of the situation. 'You have time to say goodbye.' She could have accomplished in ten minutes what took an hour – an exhausting woman. At least it gives R and K time to go swimming, and vital time to themselves.

After work K prepares Cretan chicken with crisp, bursting-with-chlorophyll broccoli and brown rice full of sweet raisins and pine nuts. With such food my strength will return soon.

Thursday 6th

Katrin: It is strange to revisit the Cottage, as we do several times a day during the week. I think, with longing, about the happy evenings we had there. I see the three of us sitting in the little armchairs, with a glass of chilled Jacob's Creek. Joan always produced delicious little nibbles to accompany the first glass: small crackers with soft goat's cheese topped with prawns and a judicious shake of paprika; anchovy stuffed olives; taramasalata or smoked salmon pâté. Each meal was prepared with all our taste buds in mind and bore the hallmark of great care and hours of work. Joan and I shared an enjoyment of trying out new recipes, leaning towards the Mediterranean and choosing light, digestible food: chicken with cracked green olives, Greek lamb avgolemono, baked aubergines stuffed with vegetables. I would usually mash the potatoes or prepare the rice, as Joan eats neither; Rory would dress the salad and open the wine. For these modest contributions we earned the accolade of 'joint effort', as though we had all shared equally in the meal's preparation just because we were lucky enough to have been the excuse for its creation.

Rory: I microwave cauliflower cheese for supper.

Friday 7th

Rory: Mum pees on my hand as I help her with her pants. 'Talk about an intimate introduction to your mother's water works,' she apologizes. She has been transcribing passages about Florida from *Next Exit Magic Kingdom* into her diary. I tell her she has better things to do with her time.

As Katrin is at work I help her to dress. An ambulance takes us to Dorset County Hospital. The driver says she joined the service three years ago after her father died of cancer. 'He went so suddenly that I couldn't reach him in time to say goodbye,' she says, topping sixty, not taking her eyes off the road.

One month ago I glanced around the waiting room and saw ill patients. Today they all look healthier than Mum. As if to underline the realization, Jan, the senior nurse, moves us to the head of the queue.

'Darling, maybe we should ask Dr Marsden about time.'

'Time?'

'So we know where we stand. I can't stay with you and Katrin forever. You have your own lives to lead. We can find out about a hospice.'

I take her hand. Our skin colour is identical.

'Are you ready, my dear?' asks Jan.

On the light boxes are a dozen scans; the insides of my mother. David Marsden stands before them, his back towards us, tapping his pen against his cheek. Jan wheels Mum's chair to his desk. She gestures for me to sit.

'How are you feeling today, Mrs MacLean?' Marsden asks.

'Reasonably well,' says Mum. 'But I've caught a cough.'

He tells us that the cancer has spread. He does not think radiation will be effective. He does not volunteer more information.

'Is it here?' she asks, touching her temple.

'Yes,' he nods. Quietly. 'I'm afraid it is.'

I hold Mum's hand again. Her eyes turn red. She doesn't cry. 'It's not a complete surprise,' she says after a moment.

'Is there anything that you'd like me to do for you?' he asks.

I don't ask about timing. I can't ask about timing.

'I'd very much like you to keep an eye on my condition, please,' she says to him. 'I'm reassured by your care.'

'I'll make an appointment for eight weeks' time,' he agrees. 'Would that be all right?'

'Thank you,' says Mum.

Jan wheels Mum into the next room for a urine test.

'Your mother looks remarkably well, considering the extent of the cancer,' Marsden tells me when the door hisses shut. He takes me to the light box. The tumour in her brain is the size of an olive; the one in her liver like a walnut. In the scans, both appear to be surrounded by shock waves; a leaden explosion pushing back the healthy tissue, cell by cell, breath by breath.

'I can't put a time on it. It could happen very soon. She may well not make the appointment in eight weeks' time. I'm sorry.'

I hesitate. 'How much should I tell her?'

'Answer her questions. If she's ready to ask them, she's ready for the answer.'

I lose my concentration. My mind clouds over. I grapple in the fog. Jan returns to guide me out of the room.

'There's something else that I need to ask but I can't quite . . .'

Jan suggests that I talk to the doctor later. Marsden sits down to write his notes. I manage to say, 'What form will it take?'

'It could take manifold forms. She could lose control of her left side again. She could suffer from abdominal swelling. She could lose interest and simply want to sleep. It depends on which of the tumours grows fastest.'

Back in the waiting room Mum chats with two nurses, sipping sugary hospital tea.

'My daughter is getting married in April,' she volunteers. 'April?' repeats the nurse.

Joan: Very fine treatment at Dorchester. Dr Marsden is a compassionate man. The cancer has spread beyond lymph to the brain. He told R afterwards, 'I can't tell what form it will take yet, but it may not be long.' He will monitor in eight weeks. Unfortunately, during our appointment the ambulance went off and the hospital couldn't reach it. A ridiculous situation as we had to wait for an hour and a half only to discover on their return they had not been busy. Fast ride back. 'Air-lifted' in carry-chair by crew upstairs to room. Relieved to be home. It is such a comfort to be here. Hugs and tears from K. Sweet call from a deeply concerned M.

Michael Frayn should have won the Booker. In *Headlong* he writes of Brueghel's ability to paint things that can't be painted – thunder, loss, the smell of the sea – as well as his extraordinary elusiveness and ambiguity. To him the artist is an absence, a ghost.

Saturday 8th

Rory: Cold, clear, sunny day. Golden light on the hill tops. Jewels in the hedgerows. Marlie arrives by train from London. Bats squeak in the station's Victorian eaves. On the way home I tell her that I've been economical with the truth. She is devastated by Marsden's prognosis.

'You can't tell her everything yet,' Marlie says after drying her eyes. 'She's so happy planning for the wedding.'

She and her fiancé, Mike – an energetic and intelligent scientist – have decided not to bring forward the date. Mum might not make it in any case.

Marlie lies on the bedroom floor, looking through gardening books. Mum has initiated a discussion on wedding colours. They may be denied the possibility of going out together to shop for flowers, dresses, the venue, but nevertheless their delight in sharing these decisions is evident. 'I adore love-in-the-mist,' she tells Mum.

'It's a summer flower, darling. I don't think it will be out in April.'

'Sweet peas?'

'Might be too forced.'

'And freesias are pretty.'

'I don't think you should have a pure white bouquet. Do you?'

Mum pushes her frame back and forth between the bedrooms for an hour, happy to be surrounded by family, determined not to use the Zimmer frame at the wedding. Until today she hadn't mentioned her presence there. Now she is wondering what she should wear on the day.

Marlie makes her coffee, buys more Fruit Pastilles, chats about a new dance company, lifts her from chair to wheeled commode.

'I feel like a jockey on his steed,' Mum declares once positioned. Her knees are bent up in front of her. 'Giddy up,' she cheers, whipping the side of the commode with an imaginary crop.

'What's the name of your steed?' Katrin asks her. We are all together in the bathroom.

'Lightning.'

I laugh out loud at the idea, as does Mum. Katrin and Marlie can't stop themselves either. They lean against the sink, unable to breathe, becoming hysterical. Downstairs Tess starts to whine.

'I wish,' gasps Mum.

In the afternoon she stops writing letters to doze in her chair, 'conserving' energy. Her throat is so sore that she doesn't want to speak. She finds it increasingly difficult to swallow pills. Marlie leans against her legs and Mum strokes her hair.

When she falls asleep I close the blind. Marlie and I ring Andrew from downstairs.

'I suppose her voice could go first,' he says from Toronto. 'I'll fly over as soon as I can.'

Katrin sets up the ironing board on the landing, looking in at her. A dozen pinpoint thrush sores line Mum's lower lip.

'I feel so sad looking at this gentle face,' she whispers to us later. 'I just want to run in and hold her. When she dies, I hope it's like that, gently, like falling asleep.'

That night, for the first time in ten days, Katrin and I close our bedroom door.

Sunday 9th

Joan: All very well with the world. M out for her walk now. R and K breakfasting before setting off on eight-mile Dorset hike and a pub lunch. Yesterday was a good day of decisions. We acknowledged that I can't manage on my own, so will give up the Cottage. At first we thought in February, but there is much to sort and an extra month will allow the luxury of time to make decisions about furniture *et al*. M will deal with my clothes. R agrees to scatter all the flower seeds about the garden in the hope they grow. I'm anxious only that I've not yet organized the family papers.

Lots of good chat with M while R and K are out; she plans to reduce to four-day working week and so visit more often. Dear call from A. Everyone sat round me on the floor and we divided the Christmas tree decorations, especially the small old wooden ones of which we are so fond.

After dinner R went into retreat watching TV as we three talked over wedding ideas, colours and flowers: lisianthus, maroons, and deep pinks for bridesmaids. K will wear her own style in dark shade, with the girls in pink/light mauve tying them together – perhaps with a sash. Long sleeves, ankle length, classic cut.

Monday 10th

Katrin: Yesterday we stepped off the map, tumbling from Bulbarrow's breezy summit down a long track through a leafless wood, following our noses. Tiny green fields flanked our descent and we threw sticks for Tess. Like us, she was drunk on fresh air, thrilled to be chasing new scents and bounding energetically about. We felt that we were the only living beings in the world. Last autumn's leaves and a light, hazy mist gave a magical hush to the little valley. Where the track broadened and levelled out, we saw a thatched cottage tucked into the tall woodland trees, serene and still in the mild January light. Nothing has ever given me a stronger sense of being out of time.

Today I brought Joan flowers from the Flower Barrow in Sherborne and arranged them in her room. We enthused together about the velvet texture and colour of the lisianthus, how their blooms contrast with the silvery green of the leaves, how the tightly furled buds look like the skirts of swirling dancers. We examined how each individual petal overlaps its neighbour and, rippling at the edge as though in motion, looks poised to swing back in the opposite direction with the next step of the dance. Never mind that they have no scent, they are so alive.

When I first met Joan, over ten years ago, she was carrying flowers, a couple of pink orchid stems, which she had brought from Malaysia where she was living with Marlie. Rory and I had only been together a short time, months, maybe even weeks, when she arrived in London for a few days' stay *en route* home to Canada. It must have been winter because I remember coats and scarves and everything drab and grey. Underneath all these layers Joan was wearing something light and floral, a skirt and shirt, visibly Malaysian, in her typical 'sweet pea' colours.

I knew from the start how important Joan was to Rory. His father had been more than twenty years older than Joan, and died when Rory was only fifteen. As the oldest of the three children, and because his mother was now alone, Rory felt that it was his responsibility to be the head of the family. Joan and he had shared financial decisions and over the years supported one another in the loving and gentle way that so characterizes the family. When he moved from Toronto to Europe, the close relationship between them continued its unswerving course. The two of them – being great letter writers – corresponded frequently no matter where they were, bridging the distance that separated them.

We ate dinner that evening in the small living room, sitting at the round table with its white chairs and pale patterned tablecloth. Two old friends were there so that

Joan and I were diluted by their company. But although we were as curious about one another as a mother and girlfriend could be, the conversation was easy and natural and I felt right away that Joan had accepted me for myself.

I remember the room's wide window admitted a soft winter light and gave a view of a large, leafless catalpa tree. But our focus was on the orchids – the centrepiece of the table – their fleshy pink lobes, illumined by the candlelight, glowing warmly, redolent of the Orient. My first impressions of Joan will forever be associated with those flowers, delicate yet strong, gracious and beautiful just like her.

Tuesday 11th

Rory: My first day away. I'm reluctant to leave home. I'm anxious that Mum might fall in my absence. Twenty minutes into the journey my mobile rings. My heart jumps. I pick up and hear Katrin's voice.

'How is she?'

'She's fine but the boiler has blown out. How do I relight it?'

Ten minutes later the train passes Castle Cary. The phone rings again.

'Would you buy a tin of coconut milk for tomorrow's curry?'

In the studio, I voice my fears. My BBC producer Mary tells me that she lost her mother last year. The week before she died Mary had to fly to Scotland to finish a programme. She instructed her mother, 'Don't you dare go before I'm back on Wednesday morning.' On Wednesday she returned to the hospital. The nurses told her that her mother was in pain and near the end. Mary sat beside her, took her hand and said, 'Go. Go now to Jerry, to Uncle Hamish. Go to Aunt May. They're waiting for you. They're all waiting for you.' A wind came up, blew through the ward, stirred the curtains and she was gone.

'Cancer is animal,' Mary tells me. 'But force of will can control it for a time.'

Late train home. In the dark bedroom I relate Mary's story. Mum doesn't respond. Her cough is deeper and drier with an unfamiliar closing wheeze. It lasts most of the night. The pastilles no longer soothe her throat.

Thursday 13th

Rory: Hard, white frost in the valley. Footprints frozen in the mud melt away as a cold drizzle begins to fall, unlike the runnels her walking frame has begun to dig in the carpet.

Twice a day a home visitor comes to wash, dress or undress Mum. Janet drives a spotted ladybird Fiat with a bumper sticker: 'Jesus loves you ... but everyone else thinks you're a wanker'. Delores – the name means sorrows – started work after her daughter was killed in a car crash. Florence Nightingale peppers her conversations with 'When you have a terminal disease ...' and 'I doubt you'll ever get strength back into those limbs ...' Her hair has been dyed an unnatural maroon colour, but not recently. Our house groans with loaned bath seats, walking frames and Pro-Pad cushions.

On Wednesday, Mum devoured a papaya for breakfast. She finished checking the page proofs of *Next Exit Magic*

Kingdom then moved straight on to reading Carol Shields' *The Stone Diaries*. She can drink from a glass again.

Today she works hard at her exercises. The physio instructs her, 'Move your arms in a big circle.'

Mum coughs with each movement.

'Now change direction. That's very good.'

'I'm showing off.'

This afternoon's carer washes her hair, then cuts it.

'Once it relaxes it will look more like you,' says Katrin.

'You mean scatty.'

Afterwards I roll up the clippings in the dust sheet. I can't bring myself to throw them away. Out of sight I shake them into an envelope and hide it in my desk.

Joan: Efficient days – Janet very helpful suggesting pine-apple for mouth sores and throat, good exercise instructions from physio Frieda and my hair cut off and well-shaped by Gisele, who works as carer four days a week, and cuts hair two nights, so she can indulge her love for horses. She has an Arab and gave her grandson a pony for Christmas. Coincidentally, her son-in-law works in Kuala Lumpur. An interesting woman with same belief as me in teaching children to be true to themselves, supporting them while they're discovering and following their own path.

M called. Coming for long weekend at end of January so R and K can go away. A wanting to come over – 'I'd come every week if I wasn't broke' – how spoilt I am with my children.

My evening walk up and down the landing's two little steps with K makes me somewhat breathless, proof that it is using different muscles and increasing oxygen intake. As I do high steps back and forth R laughs out loud at the spectacle.

'Your mother is trying to exercise, not to be a source of amusement to you,' K tells him.

'It may have taken me eighty years but I'm pleased to find what entertains you, darling,' I add.

Carol Shields' perceptive and compassionate book is imbued with wisdom and poignancy at the difficulty of simple, everyday life, but the style with frequent asides (good and pertinent as they are) is disruptive. The central character tries 'to keep things straight in her head. To keep the weight of her memories evenly distributed. To hold the chapters of her life in order.'

Friday 14th

Rory: I find Heaven and Earth in Bristol. Paula, the owner, helped to arrange Mary's mother's funeral. Mary had dressed the body in a favourite frock. She had put on a favourite hat. She had placed her mother in a cardboard coffin covered in flowers and plants brought from mourners' gardens. At the crematorium the priest said, 'I'm tempted to reach for a watering can.' There were no sycophantic undertakers; no fawning, false words of grief; no giving her up to the cold touch of strangers. The funeral was an embracing, cohesive, family farewell. Her ashes are still on the mantelpiece.

On the phone, Paula explains to me how to register a death – two doctors' signatures are required – as well as how to arrange the mortuary, coroner and crematorium certificate. At least forty-eight hours must elapse between death and cremation.

'If someone dies at home, the family may be happy to

keep the body there, but it rather depends on the weather. You don't mind me speaking like this, do you?'

I don't think I could keep Mum's corpse at home.

'Will you dress her yourself?' she asks.

'I'd find that difficult.'

'We can do it. We'll help you to do whatever you want.'

Paula asks about her height and weight. She offers me a choice of coffins – cardboard, willow or wood – and a hearse.

'Mary said that you put her mother in the back of a Passat.'

'We have a black one and a silver one.'

'Mum would prefer a silver car.'

'They're both very dignified.'

'I was thinking more about speed. She's passionate about fast cars.'

I finish writing the last two episodes of *Itchy Feet*, then stay in my study to type these notes. I've put aside my plan to write the new travel book. My world – like Mum's – is suddenly contained within these walls. Next door she opens her diary. All afternoon we write side by side, in our separate rooms. When she has filled a page, she writes in the margins. Neither time nor space is wasted. I find a grey hair on my computer keyboard.

'I think my strongest memory of you as a toddler was the time you climbed the cellar steps,' she tells me later. We have finished our omelettes. I'm lying on the carpet. Katrin is working late at Fired Earth. 'I looked up to see you crawling, halfway down the steps. There was no railing and the cellar floor was concrete. "Look at me!" you were calling. "Look what I can do!" Then you stood up on two legs.' Mum takes a breath. 'I couldn't reach you. I didn't dare to shout and scare you. So I lay down on my belly by the door and called you to me. Step by step. I grabbed you as tightly as I could as soon as you were in reach. It was the longest minute of my life.'

I wake at midnight. A minute later Mum's bedside light flicks on. Only now do I hear her moving in bed. Another minute passes and then her light is switched off. Darkness again.

Saturday 15th

Joan: M brings Mike and his teenaged son Toby – a nice lad – for fun weekend. Happy picnic lunch together in my room – village bread, ham, delicious shop cheeses. K's salads are voyages of discovery; lots of unexpected surprises on the journey. Home-made almond biscuits from Mike. Beautiful iris and pink carnations from M. All amused by my love of tennis and Formula 1 racing (especially my dislike of – but admiration for – Michael Schumacher). Reminisce about Brooklands Motor Course, the first British Grand Prix, Birkin's red 'blower' Bentley and Malcolm Campbell's Bluebird. Mike asks how I met my Andrew. I'm so bad at getting the chronology right. London 1952. Or was it 1953? He'd come to the UK to meet Fleming, and found me in the office. Three times he asked me out. Three times I refused. He was such a rascal, but with a twinkle in his eye. On the fourth attempt I agreed to meet him. Ten days later I cried seeing him off on the boat-train from Waterloo.

Now the young are downstairs. M and Mike have commandeered the kitchen. Lots of chopping for sole dish. I ask R to bring the filing cabinet down from the Cottage. He's quiet today. One of us has to go through the papers and as I'm not doing anything it might as well be me.

Sunday 16th

Rory: The house feels crowded. Katrin and I can get away for a walk but again – despite being housebound all week – I find I'm reluctant to venture far from home. I feel like an overprotective parent unable to let go of his child. I slump on the sofa and fail to read the paper. I lie in bed but can't nap. Instead, I'm listening, always listening, stretching my consciousness through both open and closed doors, trying to hold on to her, denying the inevitable.

In contrast Mum sparks with lively conviviality.

'Did you sleep well, Mike? Are you cycling to Batcombe again this morning, Toby? What do you think of a delphinium bouquet, Marlie?'

Over ginger tea she explains lightly why she won't insist on chemo or radiation treatment. 'This old body has already been through a lot.'

She chats, laughs and exercises. But by lunchtime her gregariousness leaves her exhausted, with lids heavy and speech slow. She is unable to slice her roast chicken and slops gravy on to her lap. We five eat downstairs, raising our glasses to her in a loud toast. She doesn't hear us.

When Marlie and Mike prepare to leave, she looks crumpled, leaning against the wing of her chair. I put her down for a sleep, feeling both anxious and – I'm ashamed to admit – smug; a graceless and selfish response to their care. As much as I love them, I fret that their presence upsets our daily routine. Mum needs more and more time to recover from each visit, from every telephone call. Marlie cries in the kitchen. 'I wish I didn't have to go.'

Come late evening, Mum's legs don't work at all. She stares into space, needing to be wheeled to the bathroom again. I brush my teeth. Katrin cleans her face. We exchange few words.

We are woken by her coughing at midnight, two and four. In half sleep I focus on the sound, drawing it into me, smoothing it into a blunt point, trying to use my energy to soothe it. After a moment her coughing stops. Three drunks pass beneath the window, one of them with a similar hack. I follow its sound down the street, away from Mum, until her renewed cough draws me back.

In the bathroom she says, 'I don't think we're beating this.'

I squirt morphine into her mouth for the third time that night. Her bedroom smells of perspiration and urine: pungent and biting. In our room in the dark I find tears on Katrin's cheek.

'I want to call my mother,' she tells me.

'She'll be asleep, my love.'

'I just need to hear her voice.'

Monday 17th

Rory: Heavy cloud. Slashes of silver sky between the banks. Scant light filters to earth and it stays dark under the trees until ten. Her lips and mouth are bruised red as if her blood is moving closer to the surface. Her skin is blotched as if it has thinned during sleep. We help her out of bed and she high-steps in her frame back and forth for an hour. She stoops to the left today. I cook porridge laced with heather honey while a carer washes and dresses her. Mum would prefer muesli for breakfast but it scratches her throat.

'I want to talk to Carole about hospices.'

I tell her it's too soon to talk about leaving us.

She takes my hand and probes, 'But we don't know about the timing, do we? Darling, did Dr Marsden say anything more about timing when you stayed in his office on Friday?'

'Dr Marsden told me that he cannot say how long it will be,' I repeat. How can I tell her that he expects her to be dead in less than eight weeks? I want to reassure her, not to demoralize her. I can't say 'very soon'. 'He also said that it might happen . . . quickly.'

'Because it's in the brain?'

I nod. Her look of relief surprises me.

'When the time comes, I hope that it does happen quickly. I don't want to hang around.'

Joan: CancerCare Carole is a joy. She suggests a Marie Curie nurse to relieve R and K, but R feels one is unnecessary at present. She is delighted that I'm looking and moving well and tells me that I can drink wine again (I don't mention the Christmas champagne). She wonders aloud if I should have 'a lightning flash of radiation'. I spoke to her about my decision, and about the hospice, making it clear that I do not want to remain here if it begins to affect negatively the family relationship. Carole spoke of the importance of reflection on life and on one's accomplishments. She said, 'I don't think people should remember their lives by saying "*at least* I did this or *at least* I did that". There should be no *at least*. One has to be positive about the past.'

I told her, 'How can I be anything but positive? I've been surrounded by love all my life.'

Watched Henman beat Golmard at the Aussie Open: 6–7 6–3 7–6 7–6. A positive step on a return to form.

Tuesday 18th

Rory: At six the world is cold and black beyond my window. My hollow eyes stare back at me in the glass.

'Did we tell Katrin that, if my mind goes, I want to go to a hospice?' she asks.

'The only thing that's going this morning is your memory,' I tell her.

Her nightgown is soaked with sweat again. I change her sheets, clean the bathroom, air the house and complete the radio scripts.

Katrin: These dark mornings are vile. I took Tess out for her morning walk and saw the sun coming up – at eight o'clock. Long soft clouds like rolls of dough fringed a minor constellation of brilliant, shining rafts of gold. The sky around was daubed with borrowed colour – luminous orange edging the clouds, morphing into soft pinks. The rising sun made a kind of black hole in reverse, with all the light and energy concentrated at its centre and the darkness around rapidly – yet imperceptibly – receding. It's funny how you can never really pinpoint or fix these moments of change, that they happen like the pulse of blood through your veins, as you move through time and space, as your eyes adapt to the change in light.

The spectacle made me think of Scotland and all the incredible skies I photographed during our winter living on Mull. When I got back from my walk, I asked Joan if she'd seen the sunrise, knowing how much she would love it, too. But one of the carers had been in to help her wash and her attention had been diverted from the world outside the window. She was disappointed to have missed it, so I dug out my pictures.

That year – the year we got married – we moved to Mull while Rory researched his second book, *The Oatmeal Ark*. We rented a small, west-facing croft next to Duart Castle, which overlooked a beautiful bay. There the slow, timeless rhythm of the tides punctuated the days as Rory wrote and I coiled my baskets. By then Joan was also in Scotland, not far away, living with Marlie again on her return from Malaysia. She came to see us several times and – adaptable and responsive – immersed herself as we did in the ravishing landscape.

There was never any question of autonomy when Joan stayed, of us doing anything without her – after all she came to visit *us*. We were always together, whether under one roof or out in the open – a tight family knot. We ate our meals together, went for walks together, talked about Rory's book, did our shopping together. During the day, when Rory and I were working, Joan wrote letters, read or wrote her diary. The croft was tiny, with a single living room and kitchen downstairs and two bedrooms upstairs. Yet for all this closeness, this sheer proximity – which because of our isolation could well have been claustrophobic – there was nearly always a harmonious atmosphere. We three hummed along together, in tune with our environment, sensitive to each other's needs and mindful of each other's privacy.

It was by living together like this that Joan and I got to know one another best. Our mutual love for the natural world cemented an understanding, which began first and foremost because we shared a love for Rory. On Duart Point, remote and surrounded on three sides by water, the restless mobility of the sea and sky engendered a profound appreciation for the elements, the rugged landscape they shaped and its abundance of wildlife.

When the tide was out and the bay had drained, the three

of us, dressed in thick winter woollies, scarves and rain gear, often marched across its breadth. We clambered over the lichen-covered boulders at its edge and out on to the level expanse, stepping between the thick clumps of slippery green seaweed. Groups of oystercatchers probed their long, bright orange bills into worm casts, and preened and strutted comically on their pink legs, their black and white forms reflected sharply in the shallow pools that the sea had left behind. They took wing as one, piping their loud, distinctive 'tin whistle' call. Greenshanks waded on spindly stilts, advancing jerkily through the water with heads down, sweeping them from side to side to sift the water like forensic scientists. Cautious sand-pipers, tails bobbing continuously as they fed, took off as we approached, flying low over the bay with flickering, shallow wing beats. Slowly, and unconsciously, we traced the curve of the shoreline by following the miniature furrows and ripples of the sandy seabed, which echoed its contour.

As dusk fell we heard the drawn-out cry of the curlew, solitary and familiar. We returned homewards, pockets brimming with the small trophies of our outing – razor-shells, mussels, limpets – as the light bled away and the colours became muted and monochromatic. Over the kitchen table, Joan and I pored over our field guides. Touchingly, she deferred to my ornithological judgement even though I'm no expert, knowing this was a particular love of mine. Over time I came to understand that this was more to do with tact and wanting me to feel valued than it was a real lack of knowledge. Her love of sharing and wanting others to feel included was second nature. During these times, I felt we lived together as a family almost as one does before leaving home; and because there was not then a physical house where we could all congregate, home was wherever Joan and her children met. I became quite simply – and unconditionally – a part of the family.

Wednesday 19th

Joan: R back to London to record the last *Itchy Feet* so K off work. On her drive home from the station she brings me an exquisite bouquet of fragrant pale, shell-pink roses and maroon alstromeria with a single red rose nestling at its centre. Very caring. Now she's busy varnishing the shower room walls and with household chores. The afternoon light on the hills is delicate and all the new treasures brought from the Cottage – Inuit soapstone carvings, piris and camellia in flower – make my walks more venturesome.

R home tired having interviewed John Pilger about ethical tourism and finished series. 'An exhausting day but that's how I like it.' He has booked a Ryanair flight to Genoa for weekend after next. He and K elated. Good.

Friday 21st

Rory: Overnight the constant cough – once or twice every two minutes – sprained an abdominal muscle. There are white flecks of thrush on her lower lip again – a side effect of the steroid. Mum walks before breakfast, keeping her eyes closed. I make a fruit salad of fresh melon, raspberries and tinned pineapple. Pineapple counters oral thrush.

She has been fearful of venturing downstairs, trying to come to terms with mortality by limiting her horizons. Then, a few days ago, after looking at Katrin's Scottish photographs, she began gazing out of the window. I bring from the Cottage her birdfeeder and hang it on a nearby tree. This afternoon she reads her first newspaper in a month.

'Did you hear that Dr Mahathir fired the editor of the *New Straits Times*?'

'Who, Mum?'

'The Malaysian prime minister.'

She asks to watch the Henman–Grosjean match at the Australian Open. The English seed almost loses 'because of his usual lack of concentration'.

'I don't know what his coach is thinking of; the man's an idiot.'

She updates her diary, dips into a new book, compiles a list of more items to be brought down from the Cottage. She telephones Marlie and giggles about the wedding guest list. Kleenex tissues gather in the folds of her armchair.

I order more Oramorph and protein supplement drinks. I apply for a refund of her council tax and television licence. I organize a rental car for my brother to collect at Heathrow.

'I really enjoyed today,' she tells me during her evening ramble, squeezing my hand. Her fingernails dig into my skin. 'Thank you.'

Delight animates her face, my heart lifts and I start high-stepping beside her on the landing while wanting to cry, making a game of illness, recounting a ridiculous anecdote about finding the Garden of Eden in Florida, knowing that our laughter will wear her out. Ten minutes later she looks frail again. Her skin dulls to its habitual colour. She perches her feeble body on the edge of the bed.

I help her out of an old sweater, easing it over her head, mussing her hair. I pull off her socks. I hold her glass so she can swallow a Temazepam sleeping pill. I ease her down on to her side, then on to her back and tuck the duvet under her neck. I stroke her thinning hair, then turn out the light, leaving the door ajar. When she thinks I've gone, she rubs her stomach with her fist.

Saturday 22nd

Joan: R must feel relaxed and secure about our arrangements for care as he is leaving me alone for one and a half hours to go shopping in Sherborne. I'm pleased he's taking a little time out for himself. On his return he brings me hot milky coffee and a Belgian choc – what indulgence.

Rory: To Sherborne to meet the local undertaker. Stan Blight is stepping into his car when I drive up. 'Where is the deceased now?' he asks.

'At home reading *One Hundred Years of Solitude*,' I reply.

He delays his afternoon walk to talk to me. In his office he tells me he needs a hard, blustery Saturday stomp to blow out the week's cobwebs.

'Call me Stan. No one calls me Mr Blight.'

Behind his desk hangs a violin. I ask about cost. Instead of answering me he's suddenly telling me graveyard stories.

'Once I looked after a client – a *very* pretty young graduate – who insisted on being buried with photos of her naked boyfriend.' He laughs, then adds casually, 'The truth is I've been scared of death since I was sixteen when my granny passed on. I lost my mother last year. She had cancer of the colon.'

'My mother's is in her brain. She's living with us for . . . the duration.'

'Take my advice. Don't let her die at home. It may be nice for the one who's checking out, to be all cosy and comfortable, but their family have to continue living in the house. *You* have to live all your life with the knowledge that she died in *that* room.'

I shake my head. I'm learning that dying at home brings one close to the quick of life. A painful emptiness is welling up in me like nausea, yet I feel strangely vitalized. I both hate and cherish this time, dropping habitual reticence, struggling to speak clearly from the heart. But I like Stan and his irreverent, unadorned honesty. I tell him simply, 'I need to be with her. And when she goes, I'd like you to look after her body.'

'When I die, I'll die alone. I don't want anyone else around.'

Friday 28th

Rory: My brother Andrew – who is named after our father – and his teenaged son Neal – who has snuffles – arrived from Canada five days ago, collapsing on to Mum's bed, spewing their luggage across her floor, bringing noise and life and jugs of maple syrup into the house. To celebrate we guided her downstairs that first evening. She wanted us to eat supper at a 'proper' table, and to see Katrin's finished shower room. She gripped the banister, her right hand not daring to let go, frightened of falling even though Andrew stood in front of her and I held her from behind. We applauded her descent, and – once sitting down again – settled Tess at her feet.

I've been writing for most of the week, only really seeing Mum to administer her drugs. To give Andrew some time alone with her, I took Neal to Chesil Beach. He'd never before seen the sea. We ate cod and chips on West Bay pier, looked for fossils and shopped for bagels and sliced turkey on the way home. That evening I glanced at Mum after bringing her supper on a tray. She sat with her eyes closed, her head tilted back, her hands clasped on her lap.

'I'm glad that you and I went to the sea that time in November,' she said without opening her eyes.

Andrew tried to talk about death taxes and her will. In response I retreated to my study to stare at the computer screen. Later, I apologized to him for my over-sensitivity.

'It's my problem,' he explained, shrugging. 'I hide my feelings behind details.'

He said grace before every meal.

'Thank you God for giving us this day with Mum and for keeping her free from pain.'

On Wednesday evening the new showerhead sprung a leak.

This morning Marlie arrived from London to take on the weekend's care. She, Andrew and I walked to the Cottage to review its contents. Ten years ago, Mum, determined as always to pre-empt potential friction, told us to choose our favourite paintings and pieces of furniture. Today, with her neatly typed list in our hands, we stood in the middle of the cold living room, on a family rug, looking at the escritoire, the Jacobean table, lost for words.

'Come on, let's go. This is really boring,' said Neal.

Andrew now wants the Dutch corner cabinet. Marlie would like the living-room armchairs. I'd prefer another engraving. At home we ask Mum to help us renegotiate over the grandfather clock.

'Darlings, you have to work it out,' she tells us.

After an early supper we tuck her into bed together, then take our leave one by one, before slipping away into separate worlds. Marlie calls Mike. Andrew and Neal prepare to return to Canada. Katrin and I pack our bag for Italy. We are all on our own.

Joan: A and I 'hanging out' for most of the week. He v. dear speaking of 'a charmed childhood': the old house on Highland Crescent, good education, summer holidays, relaxed welcome to his friends ('You wouldn't believe how often they asked to come and see you after school'). He spoke of my Canadian friends' loyal enquiries when they received no Christmas letters from me. R had told him exact wording of Marsden's diagnosis.

Long talk also about his new company. His faith has taught him to be accepting of God's will, thus to be less fretful, but he realizes that his whole future welfare depends on its success. He wants Neal to learn a trade so he can 'take off, travel and earn'.

I ventured downstairs for dinner – a bit wobbly at the top but with A going backwards the manoeuvre worked well. Shower room great fun with tiles and perfect painting. At supper, Neal asked me, 'Grandma, how come your feet are so calloused?' K thrilled having reserved a Genoa hotel with 'marriage bed with view of the sea'. *Una camera matrimoniale.* For me, her excitement brought back happy memories of my Italian honeymoon.

R called last ten days 'hellish'.

In Melbourne, Henman twice lost his serve and was defeated by an unseeded Woodruff. Useless.

Saturday 29th/Sunday 30th

Katrin: We dropped down on to the long, narrow coastal strip. The aircraft seemed to skim the roofs of the galleria, a series of tight tunnels that thread the ribbon of road through the mountains. A pale mantle of dust from a cement works near the airport intensified the rich blue of the sea. Everything seemed new, bright, close up; every moment leaving an indelible emotional imprint.

An hour after landing we sat nestled in a trattoria by the port, steam on the windows, the pungent smell of seafood and wine filling our nostrils. The owner took us to the kitchen where a huge basket of vegetables overflowed on to the floor: aubergines, zucchini, peppers, sedano – my Italian was coming back. Damp squalls brought in families – chattering, relaxed, laughing – until every table was occupied. Among them we drank a vibrant Pigato and ate fresh bread with small pats of butter and delicious savoury pasta dishes, mopping up the atmosphere, absorbed by it yet separate from it. The tastes, smells and humid warmth stole through me, thawing my tension, driving out the English winter.

The next day we followed a steep stony path that hugged the hillside, climbing past ancient terraces and dropping down through dappled olive groves. The hot sun warmed our backs as we panted uphill in shirt sleeves, colour in our cheeks. Cliffs plunged precipitously into an azure sea, which mirrored the sky. Small villages were perched or tucked improbably into the folds of a dizzying landscape; the bulbous cupola of a church loomed up at eye level, cats lazed in fishing boats drawn up on a minute pebbled beach. In Corniglia we discovered a tiny, hidden osteria tucked into a wall. They served us homemade *salsicce di cinghale* – wild boar sausage – with a robust local red and I wished I could stay here forever.

That evening in Portofino, a newlywed couple sauntered across the piazza, alone at last after their festivities. The bride was wearing her new husband's jacket around her shoulders and when I asked to see her dress, she shrugged it off and pirouetted gracefully, at home with her beauty and delighted to show off to strangers. Beyond her, two men with a ladder pruned the trees that lined the small square. One man mounted the steps, wielding the shears, his head vanishing beneath the tree's umbrella, while the other collected the dead wood. I glanced away for only a moment, but when I looked back, the bride, the gardeners, the moment – timeless, of the seasons, yet somehow out of time – were gone.

Rory: My mobile won't work in Italy. I buy an Italian SIM card and phone Marlie with our contact details.

February

Tuesday 1st

Rory: On our return home Mum looks radiant. Downstairs at the front door I whisper to CancerCare Carole, 'Can you tell me what's happening?'

'Your mother is amazing,' she replies, smiling. 'She looks better and better every week.'

'But she isn't getting better. The cancer is spreading. I can hear it in the changing cough. I see it in the tiredness in her eyes.'

'It must be so difficult to prepare yourself for the end and then for it not to come.'

I don't know if she's talking about Mum or me. 'She's never known that Dr Marsden gave her eight weeks to live,' I say to Carole.

'They always get the timing wrong.'

'I think she's determined to make it to Marlie's wedding,' Katrin tells her.

'When's that?'

'April twenty-ninth'

'That's three *months* away.'

'She's whipped the cancer into the corner and dared it not to come out – at least, not before the end of April.'

Upstairs Mum is winded by her walk between the bedrooms. When I climb the stairs she doesn't meet my eyes. She may have heard our whispers, though not our words.

'I should go to the hospice,' she tells me. While we were

away a Marie Curie nurse told her more about the Dorchester facility. 'So I won't be a burden on you.'

'You're not a burden, Mum.'

'But I might be hanging around for as long as a year.'

We have the possibility of making the remainder of her life bearable and contented. It's one of the jobs we are put on earth to do. But few people – because of the demands of money, career and other family – have the opportunity to seize it. I'm lucky enough to work from home, to be able to stop writing (at least until my savings run out). I have the chance to sit with my mother, to hold her hand, to be close until the hour she dies.

'We want you with us,' Katrin tells her.

Wednesday 2nd

Katrin: I made two phone calls today – one to the Bristol Cancer Care Centre for an information pack, the other about our IVF plans at Bourn Hall (of Louise Brown fame). It's already more than three years since I started trying to get pregnant. I can't bear to think with what *arrogance* we assumed we could plan it so that Rory could finish a book and I could complete my year at Camberwell. Or of the *irony* of postponing coming off the pill – by as little as a month!

Bourn Hall are holding clinical trials this year. They are going to compare the effectiveness of two types of fertility drugs, both of which have already been in use for a number of years. Female volunteers are needed who meet specific criteria (never having been pregnant being the first). Last year we applied, did the appropriate blood tests and, just before Joan became really ill, were accepted for a place on the trial. This means that they will fund the full £3,000 cost of an IVF cycle. Now we are just waiting (waiting, waiting . . .) until we can actually 'move forward'.

Of course, all our energy – and time – is now going into looking after Joan – as it should. But although Bourn Hall are very compassionate when I explain our circumstances, I don't know how long it will be before we lose our place on the trial. With this added pressure, it is agonizing to wait even a minute longer when we could be getting on with it; moving one tiny pace closer, not even to a new baby, but at least to the *possibility*, the hope, of conceiving one.

When I find myself dwelling on this, I am overcome with guilt at my selfishness, at the thought of my own needs when Joan's – and Rory's – are so pressing. And yet thinking beyond her death – for that is where I am looking – and into the heart of grief, makes my desire for a child, for new life even more urgent.

I can't really share these things with Rory right now; he needs to know that I am right beside him.

Thursday 3rd

Rory: All her life Mum has been a hoarder, not of possessions but of papers and memories. Today she starts to sieve through her files. Together we dwell on small, monochrome snapshots of her bouncing in a crib, riding a pony along the sands, in school uniform. She always seemed to be laughing, except when a stern grandmother was in the frame.

'She had a stick. It's lucky I don't have a stick or I'd be pounding it on the floor at two o'clock in the morning.'

In the matt black album are also photographs of her mother and her father.

'When Mummy was pregnant with me, she longed to eat oranges,' she recalls. She still calls her 'Mummy' because her mother died an early death and the loss prevented a part of her from ever growing older. 'Can you imagine *oranges* in 1919? Right after the Great War? My father walked all over London looking for them. I can't stand any citrus fruit.' She turns another page. 'There he is, wearing a tie on the beach. He couldn't be any nationality other than English.'

'Didn't he bring home pasta, too?' I ask.

'That was after we moved to Esher. On Saturdays he worked half-days at the bank and would go to Soho to buy fresh ravioli for supper. It was so exotic.'

Her mother had died in the dentist's chair.

'I was at school when it happened. I came home on the bus, as usual, and found my father waiting alone in the house. The poor man.'

'You were only fourteen.'

'Was I? I'm no good with figures. I think it was in 1933. Or maybe Mummy was thirty-three? I don't remember.'

When she talks her eyes often remain closed now, as if wrestling to drag memories to the surface.

'I do remember her as a gentle woman, always laughing. I also remember standing to attention when "God Save the King" was played on the wireless.'

I'm lying on the floor. My head rests on a pillow against the chest of drawers. My feet are touching hers. I say, 'You once told me that you wanted your ashes to be scattered over her grave.'

'I'd still like that. She's a bit out on a limb in Esher.'

'But won't you be out on a limb there, too?'

'I'll be with her. And two's much more friendly than one.'

'If Katrin and I ever have a daughter, we want to name her Lucy, after your mother.'

A gentle smile rises to her lips. 'I wish I'd been called Lucy. It's a lovely name. Not like Joan. Oh look, here's a photograph of Bunty.'

She natters about her friends Bunty and Margo, whose father built bridges in India. They played golf together until Mum fainted on the course.

'It's really such a silly game; you hit the ball, then walk, hit the ball, walk. I much preferred tennis, or watching motor racing.'

She talks again about weekends at Brooklands and now about Jack, the boyfriend who joined the RAF and later flew from the racecourse. He was killed in 1941.

'If he hadn't died, I would have married him. Our stories would be very different then.'

Until today she had never mentioned his name to me.

I look back in the file boxes. There are few papers from before the war. Mum's father had remarried and, when he died years later, her stepmother threw away her things.

Friday 4th

Joan: Start in on sorting files with R. He delighted by mementoes of my childhood. I was hoping to trash a lot. R talks of influence of us being much alone during his first years. On phone M and I discuss wedding flowers: pinks, purples, white for bouquets; sweet peas plus lily of the valley for table arrangements. Both crying as I so much wanted to do them.

Davis Cup GB vs Czech Republic – Henman's first service was wholly unreliable but he kept his concentration and took three sets and then the match – the first time he has won a five-setter from two down. He looked 'steely' (a characteristic he usually lacks).

Saturday 5th

Rory: 'You absolute *noodle!*' Mum shouts at Henman. England loses the final.

Sunday 6th

Katrin: I feel as though I can't breathe. The boiler is on day and night, dust is collecting on every piece of furniture, on every ledge, faster than I can get rid of it. The bathroom is always occupied – I have to 'book' to use it, and to move the commode every time I need to pee. A steady stream of visitors beats up and down the stairs: social services, CancerCare, nurses from the surgery, then at the weekend, Marlie and Mike. When we came back from Italy I found they had slept in our bed. Nowhere feels private any more.

Joan: R and K start to sort the Cottage – good that they tackle it together as R sad there on his own. K brought back foodstuffs. R working on the store room – a little at a time so no last-minute hectic rush. Later M upset that they are sorting without her, not understanding that this is just a throwing out of inessentials. She is torn trying to involve herself fully in her new family, yet balance her old family here. K also upset by misunderstanding over M and Mike sleeping in her bed.

Monday 7th

Rory: On Mum's bedside table are two pairs of spectacles, the photograph of my father, Bach's Rescue Remedy and her childhood *Reign of Old King Cole*. The hand bell and Fruit Pastilles move with her every day, from bed to chair and back again. A Christmas angel ornament perches on the bed head. Her drugs are outside her room, laid out on a chair in my study, as if they aren't hers: Thyroxine, Lansoprazole, Dexamethosone, Temazepam, Oramorph and the two laxatives.

This morning's carer – Delores – dresses her in a moss green sweater, white blouse, thermal vest and blue track trousers; ugly as hell but easier for Mum to pull down by herself. I'm distracted responding to emails so breakfast is late.

'If you have work to do, please don't worry about me,' she says.

We begin to sort the second drawer of the filing cabinet; personal letters, dated bank statements, doctor's reports. I linger over BOAC air tickets and a 'Self-Examination for Skin Cancer' card. I throw out old cheque stubs and poll tax demands.

'Why on earth have I kept twenty years of credit card receipts?' she asks me.

There's a hand-typed record of her Canadian household expenditure, dated 1971, the year that my father died. In the margin she wrote, 'The heating bills are higher than expected as the house is desperately draughty. I cannot see a chance of reducing maintenance costs until we have it in better shape – or sold.' Under Contingencies she lists $440 to replace 'rubber car hose eaten by porcupines – twice'.

In the early evening I walk the dog, light a fire and have a bath. I'm not wearing my glasses when I step out of the bathroom. I see Mum collapsed over the side of her chair, not moving. I jump forward. She sits up. She'd dropped an envelope. Later a friend, an acupuncturist, comes by the house to treat me.

'I need courage, Georgina,' I tell her.

Tuesday 8th

Joan: Sifting through my letters. I can read only a few before feeling choked up. Call M to share my success in getting out of bed unaided this week. I feel so chuffed. Now all I have to do is conquer those bloody stairs. It's the only physical effort to make me cry.

Also ask M about her choice of wedding shoes – simple, classic, wide-fitting from a dance shop. R throwing off new cold. K developing one. She brings me a delicate bouquet – sweetly scented broom (genestra) with tiny white flowers, hypericum (St Johns' wort) with just the orangey red painted seed pods, and what we think is a small-leafed euphorbia – a thoughtful surprise. Together in my bedroom R says, 'Mum, I think we're coping well now, apart from the fact that we have cancer.'

Wednesday 9th

Rory: A villager keeps two dozen parrots in his garage. Today he unlocks the doors to let in the sun and the birds squawk all morning. I open Mum's window to admit the sound of the tropics.

Dr Marsden delays Mum's eight-week check-up by a month. My annual travel insurance policy expires.

Joan: YOU CAN'T SCARE ME because EVERY NEW DAY is a GIFT.

Thursday 10th

Rory: Thursday is hair-washing day. Mum leans over the bath. Jenny, this morning's carer, pours water over her head. Shampoo. Rinse. Conditioner. Blow dry in her bedroom. Silver tendrils pulled back under black hairband. Afterwards Mum is always tired. I help her back into her chair. I lift her feet on to the footstool, feel the waning weight of her legs. I place the pink blanket, folded once, over her knees and tuck it around her hips. Hot cranberry juice by her side. I squirt Lansoprazole into her mouth and kiss her forehead. I tell her, 'I'm not surprised most faiths offer an afterlife.'

'You're sounding especially Hindu this morning, darling.'

'I feel the need to believe in it too, Mum. I couldn't carry on if I thought that consciousness ended with death.'

'Maybe it's some sort of defence mechanism but I think that somehow, in some other form or place, we'll be together again. I hope that Andrew feels the same way.'

'He believes that we'll all be united in heaven.'

'Whatever it's called, the spirit, love or God, I'm certain it lives forever. Thank you for telling me. It helps me knowing how you'll be . . . afterwards.' She puts her bowl of strawberries aside and starts to stand up. 'May I have my morning hug now?'

Joan: Stormy weather must be coming as blue tits are gathered round the feeder. Little dunnock shuffling along beneath it, twitching his wings. K stops cleaning her bedroom to stand beside me and watch. R recharges the feeder twice to prolong our entertainment. We also spot three enchanting siskins – black crown, bright yellow eye stripe, wing-bars – but sadly no parrots.

R asking over breakfast why we don't feel the need for structured religion? We believe in principles of Christianity, deep in our hearts, and follow them. Perhaps we learnt early on to be self-reliant? For us rituals are unnecessary trappings. I find walking by the sea, listening to the waves, watching the birds a more religious experience than sitting in any man-made church, however beautiful.

Friday 11th

Rory: Another good day. The wind blows away the clouds. Seagulls ride high in the clear sky. Washing dries on the line. Katrin shows Mum photographs of our Italian weekend: the curve of the Golfo di Tiguillio, the headlands of the Cinque Terre, laughter at our hotel-room window.

She starts on three thick files marked 'Letters – Friends'. 'The only problem with going through these is I realize how many people I haven't written to yet.'

At my desk I listen to the sound of her tearing pages. When I return to her room she's holding a letter from Ian Fleming to my father, recommending her as a secretary.

'Your father was very cheeky asking Fleming for a reference. By then we were both in Toronto.'

After the war my mother worked for Fleming at Kelmsley House, when he was foreign editor of *The Times*. She typed the manuscript of his first book, *Casino Royale*. I like to believe that she was the model for Miss Moneypenny.

'Fleming had an excellent secretary in New York during the war. Moneypenny was based on her.'

'Did she have red hair like you?'

'I don't remember.'

'It's not very likely.'

'Maybe there was a little bit of me in her, too. I do remember that he had another girl between us who was absolutely hopeless.'

'Did he ever try to seduce you?' I ask.

'Once he came very close, but then I think he realized that I was more use to him as a secretary. He was a good man. I wish they hadn't written those horrid biographies about him.'

While working with him she was diagnosed as having a

'weak' lung. Her doctor advised her to exchange damp London for alpine Switzerland. But by then she and my father had exchanged letters for over a year.

'It would have been so different had I gone to Switzerland or stayed with Fleming. Not long after I left Kelmsley House he moved to Jamaica to write the other Bond books. He would have asked me to come with him.'

Instead she emigrated to Canada, found an apartment in Toronto and became my father's secretary. Then she fell pregnant with me.

'I wasn't a very practical woman,' she tells me.

We spoke of her loneliness that first Christmas, when she had moved to Vancouver for my birth. At the time my father was unhappily married with a capricious and unfaithful wife.

'I just followed my heart. I knew that your father would look after me. Just like you're looking after me now.'

I bring in the washing ahead of the rain, switching on the radio while making lunch. It's been turned off for the last six weeks so as not to drown out the sound of her bell or call. Overhead I hear her walker lurching back and forth along the landing. We eat steamed broccoli with goat's cheese. At tea time I bring her milky coffee.

'I know it's a bit wicked, but do you think I could have another Belgian chocolate, too?'

When the door bell rings, Mum looks out the window. 'Oh God, it's Florence Nightingale.'

The district nurse may not be her favourite visitor but at least she brings the correct incontinence pads. While she reminisces about her last holiday, Mum closes her eyes and feigns exhaustion.

'Your mother looks very tired today,' Florence whispers to me at the front door.

'It's the time of day,' I say.

After she leaves I climb back upstairs. 'Didn't you once consider going on the stage, Mum?'

'What on earth do you mean?' There's a mischievous glint in her eye.

'I'm surprised that you didn't start moaning for dramatic effect.'

'I thought that might be gilding the lily.'

Saturday 12th

Rory: 'I'm a company director,' Marlie tells us over the phone. She and Mike are building a virtual cemetery to 'keep memories alive'. Visitors to their website will be invited to register the names of departed family members and friends, and to share their recollections with others. The intention is to give the bereaved a focus for their memories and help them to deal with grief.

Monday 14th – Valentine's Day

Rory: Yesterday didn't exist. Katrin and I went next door for Sunday lunch and came back seven hours later.

'Considering the amount of vodka you've drunk you look remarkably well,' Mum tells us.

Then we polished off a bottle of wine in front of the TV.

Come this morning my head is vacant. I lie on the floor of Mum's room, lights off, staring into space. Neither of us has the strength to sort files. When her eyes are closed, I steal glances at her, trying to memorize her features. Around midday I manage to make it to the Cottage to sort through her garden tools. I throw out blue slug pellets and give trays of seedlings to her neighbours. Katrin returns from work to find me back on the floor, talking to Mum in the dark.

We ask her again if she'd like to come downstairs for supper. She bites her lower lip.

'If I hold on to your shoulders and not the banister I might be able to get around that corner . . . tomorrow.'

Katrin cooks us piperade – peppers, tomato, garlic, basil, eggs. She and I watch a *Horizon* special on disease. The programme suggests that cancer may be a virus, and contagious. We decide not to tell Mum.

At ten I pack for London and Katrin cleans the kitchen floor. 'I can't get on top of this dust,' she says.

Half an hour later while I brush my teeth and Katrin discusses cuticle cream with her, Mum has a coughing fit.

'Jesus,' she curses, wincing in pain as I swing her legs into bed. 'Sorry. I'll be fine tomorrow. Night night.'

Tuesday 15th

Katrin: Skies pleated with pale grey clouds. A whiff of snow in the air. In the clearings, jet streams like long threadworms. A milky, glareless white spills from a mute sun, the edges of its disc indistinct.

Joan had been looking really well. She was taking care of her appearance and was her neat and tidy self again. Only her thick green oversocks, which she wears as her poor feet are too swollen for shoes or slippers, give her away. When she walks they slowly work their way off her feet and trail along the floor, a bit like a baby's do when they are at the crawling stage. It makes me feel really sad.

Then last night we were woken by the sound of her banging the wall with her knuckles. Her head had slipped off and beneath the pillow. She couldn't move her limbs or reach the bell. Brown phlegm stained the sheet. We eased her swollen feet over the side of the bed and her legs went rigid. Her heels were raw from lying in bed. To keep her warm we dressed her – sweater, track trousers, those socks – and walked her to the toilet but she was too tense to pee. Her face was chalk white.

Rory cancelled his London meetings. The doctor came at nine. Joan's hand locked on his shoulder as he examined her. He found a torn muscle below her ribcage.

'If it hurt, why didn't you take more Oramorph?' he asked her.

Sometime later I drag myself out of the house to walk Tess. So tired. She halts in her tracks and lifts a paw for me to inspect. I check for thorns but find nothing. She trots homewards again, happy for the attention she's been missing.

Wednesday 16th

Rory: Her bell rings. I sit bolt upright in bed, shot out of a dream. I call into the darkness, 'I'm coming.' Katrin swears.

Mum smells of illness again. 'Jesus,' she says again as I help her to her feet. At first she doesn't walk. Instead she stands in the frame and lifts her legs up, left right left right, like a broken clockwork soldier. 'I'm so thirsty.' I lift the glass so she can drink. Then we find our way to the bathroom. I sit at my desk to wait and stare out at the night.

When I help her into bed she bites her lip. 'I have to lie straight,' she tells me, snaking sideways across the mattress. 'Help me to lie straight.' She winces again as I centre her head and shoulders on the pillow. She doesn't cry.

In the morning I ask her too many questions: 'Can you finish your breakfast now? Would you like a cup of soup? Shall we try the comfortable armchair?' She just shakes her head, unable to answer, unable to see through the morphine haze. She walks only once to the bird window. The car breaks down on Katrin's drive to work. Malcolm the mechanic can't fix it until Friday.

The robin is blown off the birdfeeder, jackdaws are swept from the chimney pots. The sunshine gusts through her room. I watch the light glance across her face and – as time and morphine ease her muscle pain – she begins to reminisce about her first arrival in Canada. She tells me that her ship docked late in Québec City and that she and my father ate the lobster thermidor dinner for breakfast. He took her by train to Toronto and, later, when she was pregnant, on to Vancouver.

'It's *so* long ago.'

'Not that long.'

They went for walks in Stanley Park, watched the seals at Vancouver Zoo until my father returned east. Old Toronto was too intolerant – and he was too well known – to condone or even acknowledge a love child. She had no friends from ante-natal class to share with. No old schoolmates to take her to the hospital. Her only company was the woman in the next room who had a four-year-old child of her own.

'What was her name?' asks Mum.

She was alone when I was born. My father sent express packages of baby clothes for 'his little seal'. After two months he brought us back to Toronto and bought her a compact bungalow on Chaplin Crescent. She and I lived there alone for the first years, apart from local society. He came by every morning as the divorce was negotiated.

'We lived in our own little world. It was so hard on your father.'

Mum stops speaking again. She lays her fingers against her throat as if to soothe its rawness. In the fading sun her hands appear ridged and calloused like a schoolboy's papier-mâché relief map. She coughs a toad-like croak and asks for more morphine. It's only three hours since her last dose.

'But your side seems to be getting better,' I say.

'It's not my side. It's my back. I don't know why my back's hurting.'

I make her hot chocolate. She closes her eyes for a moment. I sit next door to wait.

Thursday 17th

Rory: 'Honey in the morning, honey in the evening, honey at supper time. Be my little honey, and love me all the time.'

Bright, misty day. Molecules of rain and light are equally dispersed in the air. Mum has an old song in her head.

'Your father used to sing it to me. It was one of his favourites.'

I'd like to surprise her with a copy of it. A friend at the

BBC finds 'Honey' – recorded by the Andrews Sisters – in the sound archive.

'It has a quite different lyric to the one you quoted,' my friend tells me, exposing memory's magical act of self-deception. 'But Andrew Sis sung a song with the right words called "Sugar in the Morning".'

'Sugar in the morning, sugar in the evening, sugar at supper time. Be my little sugar, and love me all the time.'

Joan: R cancelled his plans again because I was in a lot of pain with torn muscles on left-hand side under ribcage. We find first picture of him taken in Vancouver hospital.

'We are praying for you,' says A from Canada. All excited about coming over in April. Just short talk to M as feeling pretty exhausted.

CancerCare Carole brings a posy of snowdrops and tells me, 'It's difficult being a patient. Are you fed up yet?'

Central heating breaks down.

Kate Atkinson's *Behind the Scenes at the Museum* is a remarkable first novel, written in what appears at first to be a haphazard fashion – but is cleverly tied together at the end. Set in York, the theme of history, both of city and a large family, is strong. Narrated by Ruby from her conception to her mother's death.

Friday 18th

Katrin: Joan has been living with us for seven weeks now. Today she's sorting papers again; whole sheaves of A4 – a lifetime's rubbish – are being pitched out into big black bin bags. There is a renewed sense of busy-ness here; it's as if Joan is on a mission.

As well as giving herself a purpose, she is tying up loose ends, leaving life with no unfinished business. She is remarkably practical about what she should (or in this case shouldn't) leave behind, both literally and metaphorically. I admire how equable Rory, Andrew and Marlie are, too, in this regard – they have obviously inherited this from Joan. She is wise to have sorted out the main part of her estate already so that nothing can come in the way of good relations, and so that her legacy will only be positive. It's dreadful how often families fall apart fighting over the will, over the material things, which displace grief and your loved one.

She's sorting everything from newspaper clippings and tax returns to her most precious correspondence, her letters from her husband, Andrew. She keeps this bundle under her chair, and reads them privately – and often.

Whenever anyone arrives to see her, Joan insists, 'We're getting there,' in answer to their enquiries about her health. I'm finding this delusion one of the hardest things to deal with. When she moved in, we prepared ourselves for the end, and it's been difficult to adjust our expectation.

Saturday 19th/Sunday 20th

Rory: What to do with four crystal decanters? An incomplete willow tree dinner service? A canteen of mismatching silver? Marlie and Mike are helping to sort the Cottage. We box the glass and tableware. I deal with the books. They're full of pressed flowers. We find my grandfather's silk handkerchiefs, folded between tissue paper. The table linen, too, is separated by sheets of tissue. We work quickly. I don't dawdle or meet Katrin's eye. She and Marlie divide the clothes into three piles: to keep, to sell, to give to the charity shop. Stray hairpins fall out of cardigans. Time-thinned bath towels go into the rubbish. We'll try to flog the cooker, refrigerator and bed. The personal memorabilia is more difficult: a child's Victorian tea cup, a sailor's pocket compass with its glass cracked, a ceramic Loch Ness monster inside which is a note in Mum's handwriting, 'Given to me by Rory on his first trip to Scotland'. At the bottom of the dower chest are baby booties, a child's jacket and six smooth white pebbles from a Dorset beach. Under her bed is a stack of my prep school drawings.

We lug down the High Street pot plants and frying pans, bedside tables and a rug. At home we find that Mum has been coughing for an hour. She didn't telephone because she didn't want to bother us. Katrin runs upstairs to dispense the Oramorph.

Later, Mike and I shift the furniture: the campaign chest comes into our bedroom, two chests of drawers and a rug are loaded into his vehicle for London. So Mum need not come downstairs, her old dining table is set on the landing and laid with family silver and crystal. We carry roast lamb, baked potatoes, vegetables and wine up from the kitchen. Mum eats two slices of meat and drinks a glass of Jacob's Creek. Then, as I serve the ice cream, her energy melts away. Her shoulders droop and her head tilts back. Deep circles appear under her eyes. She dozes in the chair while Mike – laptop on table – takes us on a tour of their new website. He and Marlie plan to send promotional mouse mats to hundreds of British undertakers. Their cemetery has no interns, yet.

All afternoon, Mum is short of breath. She speaks little, so as to rest her throat, but the cough is persistent. She naps for an hour then shuffles between the upstairs rooms, her lower jaw trembling, her brow knotted in concentration. A week ago I was certain that she'd live until the wedding.

Joan: How can one family have so many chairs? We are surrounded by them. The men emptied my loft, K transplanted my favourite plants and M – who is rather quiet – sorted my clothes, bringing down shoes, some of which, to my relief, fit. We will try on the dresses and skirts later (only full gathered waists may go around my tummy). Amazed how much could be crammed into Mike's van. When they reached London, M phoned to say the carpet was down and looked lovely (it will make her feel v. at home to have some of our things). Indigestion/gas could be caused by steroids. Reading Alan Bennett's *Writing Home*.

Wednesday 23rd

Rory: A flush of visitors: Mum's neighbour appears this morning, her oldest friend calls from Canada to ask if she can come next month and Katrin's parents arrive from Kent this afternoon. Katrin cooks risi bisi for supper but Mum won't eat rice or bacon. I'm graceless with Katrin and our guests, irritated by the shift of attention away from Mum. I bake her cod fillet on shredded leeks, the kitchen pungent with the whiff of burning martyr. She eats only half, leaving the rest for lunch tomorrow.

Monday night brings a hard frost. On Tuesday Katrin

and I escape to walk in the hills above Sydling St Nicholas. Her parents are on duty. The mobile is in my pocket. We talk about money. My share of the inheritance – pooled with my sister's – might buy a small flat. For years I've worried about having no money. Too soon I'll have a little. What difference will it make to my life? I'll be less worried, and less rich. The icy clods of ploughed earth crumble under our feet.

Mum watches tennis most days. Rusedski wins his match ('A dull game; it's more exciting watching the chaffinches on the feeders'). She takes her morphine and naps in the chair. Katrin joins her parents for another amble. After each match I help Mum on to her feet and we toil along the hall to stand together at the bird window.

I know I am lucky. Underneath the acute, extended pain of dying, there's an immense uncomplicated love between us. Her illness hasn't made her turn on me. The brain tumour hasn't promoted some terrible character change that, after a lifetime of devotion, suddenly makes me question our whole relationship. I'm supported by family and friends. Yet instead of counting my blessings I feel angry, betrayed, alone.

In bed Katrin curls into my arms. 'I'm so depressed,' she says.

'Why, my love?'

'All this time I've been worrying about your Mum, about Joan, Joan, Joan. Now – with their visit – I can't stop thinking of my parents. *My* mother will die, too.'

Joan: Why is everyone coming to see me? Do they think I'm about to pop off?

Thursday 24th

Rory: At 1.00 a.m. Mum rings her bell. She forgot her sleeping pill. Three hours later I realize that I am still awake, waiting until her bell rings again. When it does, I pull on my dressing gown and stagger along the hall. I help her to the edge of the bed. Her sheets are uncreased. If she were to vanish now her feather-weight would have left no impression. I reach for the walking frame. We shuffle to the loo. She lifts her hands above her head as if to drain herself. Back at the bedside her fingers feel for a Fruit Pastille. Black is her favourite flavour. Under the lamp her swollen knuckles are thick knots in slender ivory branches. I guide her head back on to the pillow. She grits her teeth but the pain is easing. I fold the duvet over her and turn off the light.

At 4.45 a.m. a wrenching, feral cough rises from her diaphragm. I forgot her morphine. While filling the spoon I spill three drops on the carpet. 'Sorry, darling,' she says, but it's my fault. On my way back to bed I pass Katrin at our bedroom door. We catch each other's hand, our fingertips brushing in the night. We sleep. I wake before the alarm, help Mum into her chair and make a sandwich to eat on the train.

8.00 a.m. Carer arrives. 8.10 a.m. I leave home. 8.30 a.m. Swim thirty lengths in Sherborne pool. 9.13 a.m. Depart Sherborne for Waterloo. Lunch with publisher. Pick up Katrin's repolished engagement ring. To Hayward Gallery for Panamarenko exhibition, then drinks at a retirement party at Bush House. 7.35 p.m. Depart Waterloo. 9.37 p.m. Katrin collects me at Sherborne station. 10.05 p.m. Reheated chicken supper. 11.00 p.m. Bed. 1.15 a.m. Her bell rings.

Katrin: Mum and Dad left today. Their visit gave Rory and me the chance to get out for a long walk together (on the downs where we could get some height and a view). More importantly, I felt reassured to have them here. Their care and support felt so *vital*, so soothing; in some ways I was a child again. I could wrap myself in their love and feel the simple, everyday familiarity of being together: pruning and tidying the garden with Dad, visiting the garden centre to buy a climbing rose, chatting to Mum, going for a walk together. It was such a relief to have them here.

Joan: As his father would have been, R is very taken with Panamarenko, a Belgian inventor-cum-sculptor: born 1940, surrealist in tradition, steeped in neo-Dada movements of 1950–60s – dead-pan whimsy. At the heart of his work is the idea of an improbable object erupting into life. 'It was as engagingly dotty an exhibition as I can remember.' Spiritual mentors: John Tinguely, Roland Emett, Heath Robinson.

Friday 25th

Rory: *Wanderlust* wants an article on the role of chance in travel. I write, 'The journey – with its beginning, middle and end – is a convenient metaphor for life.'

Yesterday Mum rediscovered coffee ice cream and today she eats three bowlfuls of it. After dinner we read downstairs. Me: *On the Road*. Katrin: *The English Home*. Above us the bedroom door opens, the frame rumbles down the landing, water runs into the sink.

'Rory, I don't feel right.'

Upstairs she is bent double, blood rushing to her head. Her left hand grips the rim of the basin.

'I can't let go.'

I pry free her hand.

'I'm dizzy.'

Katrin brings a chair. 'Sit down, Joan. Sit.'

I've been adjusting her medication. The morphine needs to be cut back to ease her constipation even though every decrease makes her cough worse. I've also been reducing the steroids. When she came home from hospital she was on eight milligrams a day. In her second week I alternated between seven and eight milligrams a day. By the third week she was down to seven milligrams. Dexamethasone reduces the swelling in the brain but the body builds up resistance to it. It lifts blood sugar and brings on the risk of glaucoma as well. We need to trim her prescribed dosage now so it can be increased later, when she'll most need it. This week she has been on five milligrams. I forgot to give her the fifth pill after lunch. I curse my forgetfulness.

'I feel so wobbly. I just need to catch my breath.'

Katrin, standing behind the chair, meets my eye. We wheel her back into her room, helping her into the armchair. As I tuck the blanket around her, Katrin massages her legs.

'I'm all right now. Thank you.'

'I love you,' Katrin tells her. 'We want you here with us.'

We almost went out to a movie this evening. We almost left Mum alone. Later she snores. At least I remembered her sleeping pill.

Saturday 26th

Rory: Porridge and honey. Morphine and steroids. All morning I listen to the sound of her tearing up her life, or at least the first draft of its record. I bring her the last drawers of letters. She sits bolt upright in her golden armchair, surrounded by teetering stacks of files.

'I'm throwing out correspondence that I thought was vital two months ago.'

There are brown envelopes marked 'Family: winter 1989' and 'Friends: 1999'. Her files are organized by name, place and year. Letters and their responses are clipped together. There are notes of condolence for my father, reams of book reviews and dozens of diaries. Dollar bills and old pound notes are secreted among the papers.

'I hid them to have the thrill of rediscovery later.'

I take away another black bin bag and return with the last Belgian chocolate and a milky coffee. She hands me her love letters from my father. 'Do read them.'

I open an envelope. I see the words 'darling', 'Little Poodles' and 'all my love'. The young hearts drawn in red pencil and eager xxx kisses are almost fifty years old.

'I can't, Mum. It feels intrusive.'

'They're here for you when you want to look.'

The bestial cough claws away all day as if its nails are scratching at her throat. Katrin brings home violets. Baked potatoes for supper. I need a drink.

Sunday 27th

Rory: Windy and cheerful morning. White sheets snap on the washing line. Chubby thrushes hunt for worms. Mum sorts through her gift box, asking me to wrap and post birthday presents months in advance.

'Dearest Mary: This jigsaw puzzle was to be your next hostess gift. Probably best that I send it to you now.'

She hurries to the window when Katrin spots a greenfinch. I stand with them plotting to move trees and shrubs, thinking about the garden in one or two years, knowing that she will never see its changes. This is her last season.

'Mum, isn't December the best month for transplanting trees?'

'Not before.'

'I want to take out that eucalyptus when the sorbus grows.'

'The eucalyptus does hide the neighbour's roof. And the sorbus isn't evergreen.'

'Do you think that the lavender is too big?'

'Never cut it back to the bare wood. It has a limited life.'

She battles with her own limited life by 'getting on'. At the bathroom door she pauses to point at her face towel on the floor.

'I don't want to bend down, darling. Would you mind picking it up for me?'

'How did it get there?' I ask.

'I swept it off as I flew by with the Zimmer frame.'

Rip hack rip burp rip hack rip burp; she coughs and passes gas as another rubbish bag is filled.

Katrin: When I came upstairs Joan asked me whether I was having a relaxing afternoon. I replied that I was doing a few small chores, then hurried away. I couldn't tell her the truth, that I was sorting through her china, that we're selling her blender at a car-boot sale, that we are dispensing with the surplus accretions of her life.

Joan: Yesterday Kafelnikov beat Rusedski in two straight sets at Axa semi-final. The Russian played superbly for the first set, then a lapse, then back to form. Today I watched Marc Rosset's spectacular defeat of him in straight sets. Rosset, a v. tall man who is remarkably quick despite his size, was made angry by Kafelnikov's condescending smile. His service was exemplary. A delight to see him enjoy his victory.

R receives a bereavement card from the hospital's dotty occupational therapists. 'We're so sorry to hear of the loss of your Mum.' Last week he left a message asking them to take away the unused bath-seat. Now they assume I am dead.

Monday 28th

Rory: Clear, cool morning. Bright blue sky. Three daffodils are out in the garden. I wake convinced that the last months have been a dream. Mum isn't ill. There is no cancer. I bounce into her bedroom and propose driving her to the coast for a walk along Chesil Beach. The suggestion defeats her, reducing her to tears.

Tuesday 29th

Rory: 'Try to have a little lunch.'
  'The spinach doesn't taste of anything.'
  'At least the egg.'

'I can't stomach anything more. I feel so bloated.'

Mum is off her food, apart from coffee ice cream. She no longer enjoys asparagus soup. She tells me that she's 'sick to death' of fruit tea. Even her favourite stand-by – baked cod – has lost its appeal. She may be accepting of death but she is battling against the idea of dying.

'There's so much I have to do,' she tells us, too concerned with her sorting.

'Not that much, Mum. There's lots of time,' I lie.

'You should take it easier, Joan,' says Katrin.

To 'get her blood moving' she performs the high step up and down the hallway, burping without stop for ten minutes.

'I feel so crushed up in the middle. It must be indigestion,' she says.

I nod in response.

'And my sides are hurting.'

'Your sides?'

'As if I've pulled the muscle again.'

'It could be the cough,' I suggest, not believing my own words.

'Never mind. It'll iron itself out.'

'Do you want to sit down?' I ask twenty minutes later.

'I can't. I need to stretch my stomach. It's best that I keep walking.'

She stops only for tennis and ice cream. I place a small electric heating pad on her lap. She sits with her arms held above her head, trying to stretch her distended stomach, but she can't find a comfortable position. She jerks herself to one side and moans into her cupped hands. The blood drains out of her face.

'It'll be all right once the heating pad warms up,' she sighs to reassure us.

I close the door on her and Rusedski. Katrin and I huddle

together in my study. Katrin whispers to me, 'She's so pale.'

'I know.'

'It might not be very long.'

'She can't go now. I'm too exhausted.'

Joan: Very tired and weepy tonight – to bed just before 10 p.m. so disturbed sleep – R feels I've been overdoing the paper sorting so will skip it tomorrow. Concentrating on M's wedding is my priority.

March

Wednesday 1st

Joan: 'All of us, all of us, all of us
    trying to save
    our immortal souls, some ways
    seemingly more round-
    about and mysterious
    than others.'

Thursday 2nd

Rory: Mum is reading Raymond Carver's poetry. She doesn't want to talk to me. Time hangs on my hands. I fill the birdfeeders as sparrows wait in the bushes. I look up and see her watching from the bedroom window. She smiles and waves. I'll never again look at that window without seeing her there. Suddenly it's six o'clock and I've achieved nothing.

Friday 3rd

Rory: Gusting winds and heavy rain. The Wriggle rises four feet in the night and threatens to break its banks. The floods delay the carer. Alone in the rain I run up the High Street, carrying the kettle and tea. The removal van arrives at nine. The contents of the Cottage are split into three. Furniture is wrapped for Toronto, packed for London or trucked to my house. Pieces that have been together for all my life are separated. On the back of the oak dresser, previous movers have written in chalk 'MacLean: Highland Crescent', then 'Russell Hill Road', then 'England'. The men move quickly, in a fleet-footed ballet of padded cardboard and bubble wrap, yet I will them to work faster. The job takes four hours, including two tea breaks and the delivery of my inheritance. Then the men are gone and I walk back home.

Saturday 4th/Sunday 5th

Joan: Slept until 5 a.m. then dozed – it is a long two hours until seven.

Rory: I wake to find Mum tearing up old recipes.

'I couldn't sleep so I thought I'd make myself useful.'

Her wastepaper basket is full of seafood menus and a bulging green file labelled 'Leeks'. The heating pad is curled around her waist. She's in pain today.

Macaroni pie.

Braised celery.

Eggs en cocotte with asparagus.

'This torn muscle is a real set-back,' she tells me, reaching above her head and spilling a dozen chocolate pudding recipes on to the floor.

'It's still hurting?' I ask while gathering her clippings.

'Quite a bit.'

Caesar salad.

Vegetarian moussaka.

I'm sure that her pain isn't muscular, that the cancer has spread from her liver.

'Darling, aren't people who have an illness from which . . . from which they're unlikely to get much better, supposed to be profound and contemplative?' she asks. 'I keep thinking that I should be having Great Thoughts about the meaning of life and all that. But nothing like that occurs to me.'

'Are you feeling a sense of incompleteness?'

'Maybe.'

'You're not burdened with unfinished business, Mum. You've always followed your heart, and look at everything you've achieved. You showed us how to love, how to be true to ourselves. In a way, you've been having Great Thoughts all your life. Maybe that's why there's no need for profundity now.'

She takes my hand and says, 'After all the books I've read these past weeks, I've been expecting the heavens to open and God to speak to me.'

'Has He turned up?'

'Not yet.'

Curried nut loaf.

Spiced pears in cider.

Guacamole.

Marlie and Mike are down for the weekend. They have to see the registrar and finalize details for their wedding ceremony. Marlie lies on the bed, discussing with Mum the reception menu and a visiting group of Russian scientists, while Katrin makes goat's milk yoghurt. It curdles. I grill plaice, and burn it. Then Katrin and I drink too much and argue about nothing. I overreact to the disagreement.

'Can't you accept that couples argue, even when they're not under pressure?' she snaps at me.

'For me, it's a failing.'

'So to you, I'm a failure.'

'A failing of communication.'

During the night we turn away from each other. In the morning Marlie looks after Mum. In bed, behind a closed door, Katrin tells me she was envious of the ease with which Marlie and Mike were able to go for a pub lunch yesterday.

'We can't be spontaneous anymore. We have to plan everything.'

'Let's go for a walk by the sea this afternoon,' I suggest.

'Will Marlie be able to cover for us?'

After lunch we drive to Durdle Door. We chase up the cliffs, lie in the sun, reach out toward the far, silver horizon.

'Last night I felt you were beginning to crack,' says Katrin to the sky. 'I thought that I have to get you out before you go loopy.'

'I was just tired. Tired and drunk.'

Monday 6th

Rory: Not a great day. The Escort refuses to start. I call the *Blackmore Vale Magazine* to sell Mum's beds and, in the middle of placing the ad, their booking system crashes. Finally, my Macintosh shuts itself down. Can grief and anxiety be transmuted into starter motors and computer software?

I'm overwhelmed and undermined, on edge and exhausted. My house is full of used beds, BBC period drama DVDs and hundreds of chewed pencil stubs. I spend the morning sorting my office, trying to create a calm centre, combining Mum's stationery with my own. I now have four staplers and nine rulers. At lunchtime Katrin finds me hunched over three bags of foreign coins, separating Malaysian ringets from Canadian loonies. Illness is emotional but it generates a great deal of edgy frustrated boredom as well.

Instead of eating lunch, Mum lies down to stretch herself. On a Post-it note I record her symptoms – 'burping, pain in side, indigestion and waning hunger, sweet tooth, thrush, broken sleep, slowly slipping'. CancerCare Carole arrives and feels her abdomen. The tumour in her liver is pressing against her diaphragm, causing the deeper cough, as well as against her stomach, making her burp and reducing her appetite.

'I know it's in my brain,' Mum says. 'I know it's in the lymph system. So I figure that it's whizzing around everywhere.'

Carole outlines the options. We increase either the morphine or the steroids. 'But I don't really want to give you more steroids quite yet.'

We settle on fifty per cent more morphine.

'Thank you for trying to make me comfortable,' Mum tells her. She accepts that nothing else can be done.

Afterwards I take her hand and tell her that she is being brave.

'I'm not being brave. I'm just not thinking.'

Katrin: I'm trying to pick apart my feelings and take a step back from the emotional ricochet of these days.

It is hard to share a house with someone who is dying, someone you love. As well as being a dearly loved mother, Joan is already the object of our grief. I don't know where to put such intense feelings when we cannot escape them, when we are nearly always together – they pervade every corner of the house. I can't prise Rory from Joan's side, though I know how necessary it is. His love for her has become over-protective, all consuming. He has turned caring for his mother into a new *raison d'etre*, bringing with it the same obsession that drives his writing.

Tuesday 7th

Joan: An exciting bird morning with greenfinches and a single, chubby coal tit. Beyond the amiable gathering, K is working hard in the garden, transplanting the Cottage plants: geraniums under the birch, hellebore near the daffodils. R prunes the rose less successfully. In London, M, who takes the day off work to receive furniture, is also in her garden, putting in bedding plants. Touching letter from Mike saying how proud he is to be marrying her.

Rory: In my dream there are drops of blood on Mum's pillow. In her dream Katrin sees a date and thinks, 'Joan won't live until then.' When Katrin's grandmother died, she simply stopped breathing. Her passing was so gentle, so lacking in drama, that Katrin's mother – who was sitting by the bed – hardly noticed the change. She went looking for a nurse to ask what was the matter.

Wednesday 8th

Katrin: Today we cleared the last few things out of the Cottage. We pulled the glazed door across the bristles of the doormat and turned the key in the lock for the last time. The finality of the moment wrong-footed me. Suddenly I felt as if I was in a children's story. I know that the magical walled garden exists but the door to it has vanished.

It is here at the Cottage that I sat at the small blue kitchen table, crying because I longed for a child. It is here that Joan took my hands and told me that she knew it would one day come true because she had heard his laughter in her dreams.

Thursday 9th

Rory: Mum tries to hold on to patterns, marking her day with the birds' routine. Flocks of passing starlings upset the order, as do the quarrels of sparrows, which descend at all times, in a frantic surge, on to the feeder.

'Look, a brimstone butterfly,' Mum calls down to us as we sort another car-boot box. 'The first one I've seen this year.'

Like the sparrows, we are in and out all day, but tie ourselves to a soup lunch, tea-time ice cream and omelette supper. I measure out life in spoons of Dexamethasone and Oramorph.

'What time is your girl coming tonight, Mum?' I ask every afternoon.

Every third Thursday she has her hair cut. Once a month her blood sugar is tested. Glandosane synthetic saliva relieves the dryness of her throat in seconds. A tube of Fruit Pastilles lasts thirty-six hours. There are pink blossoms on the prunus. I wind the bedside alarm clock.

Saturday 11th

Rory: On Friday, Mum's oldest friend, Margaret Ann, arrives from Canada for the weekend. Her son and I used to play together with plastic dinosaurs. She sits in the green bedroom, talking of children, summer cottages and Broadway costume design. Mum coughs and brightens through the morning. I produce some lunch, and can hardly get a word in to ask if they'd like more salad. They drink coffee and chat through nap time.

'I'd call them puff sleeves, with a fullness in the shoulders.'

'I imagine dancers doing it more than actors.'

They talk all today as well, laughing and watching the Australian Grand Prix. Mum shows off her childhood photo album.

'Remember I mentioned "combinations"?' she says, pointing at the snapshot of a happy toddler. 'Here I am, aged three, wearing a combination.'

'Don't you look adorable? I love your haircut.'

Margaret Ann's visit enables me to get out of the house. Again I feel relieved, and vacant. I snack on toast. Finish a year-old box of Frosties. Read another chapter of Kerouac. I can't work. I write only these few lines. I think of time wasting, and find myself imagining ahead to the vacuum after death. 'Vacuum: space entirely devoid of matter; absence of normal or previous content of a place, environment, etc.' In a week or a month the light green room will be empty. Where today I listen for Mum to call my name, there will come no sound. Where I hear the scrape of her spoon on a bowl, there will be silence. Where now I have no time, I will have too much of it.

In the afternoon I leaf through another box of her books, finding well-thumbed copies of *The House of Spirits*, *British Garden Birds* and Fromm's *The Art of Loving*. In pencil Mum has underlined: 'To be concentrated means to live fully in the present, in the here and now, and not to think of the next thing to be done.' I didn't know that Mum had read Fromm. I don't know where or when she bought the book. 'The ability to be alone is the condition for the ability to love.'

Late afternoon, a gloomy stranger telephones in response to my ad in the *Blackmore Vale*.

'Is the Z-bed still for sale?' he asks. 'Would it be convenient for us to come by now? We happen to be in the area.'

He wears a dark suit and drives a black, windowless van. His beard is neatly trimmed. His gangly assistant is equally sallow and sombre. They buy Mum's rollaway bed.

'This is our third visit to the village this month,' says the man.

'Were your previous calls on . . . business?' I ask.

'March is always a busy month.'

The assistant picks up the bed by himself. I offer to help him but he calls over his shoulder, 'I'm all right with it, thanks. I used to be a removals man.'

'Now he's in a different line of removals, if you catch my drift,' explains the older man, with a wink. I've never seen an undertaker wink. 'Put it next to the stretcher, Ken.'

Sunday 12th

Rory: Margaret Ann packs to return to Canada. While I take her to the station, Katrin carries the lunch tray upstairs. Mum is in the bathroom.

'I'll just leave your salad here by your chair, Joan,' she calls through the door.

'I thought lunch was going to be another twenty minutes,' snaps Mum. 'Now it's here and I'm not ready.'

Later she barks at me, 'I don't want to read something second rate.' I'm trying to help her to find a new book. She's rejected Cormac McCarthy, Charles Frazier and Rebecca Wells. 'I don't want to waste my time.'

When she settles on Naguib Mahfouz, I turn away to oil the squeaking hinges of her bedroom door. A white stone doorstop catches my eye. Suddenly, horribly, I want to throw the rock at her.

Monday 13th

Katrin: The strain of these last months is beginning to show on Rory. I'd always wondered how he would cope with Joan's death, and privately dreaded it. But of course this is different from the sudden, dark bereavement I'd imagined. It's much more complicated and real.

One thing I had not anticipated was that Rory would have to stop writing – and how this would affect him. I'm not talking about the loss of at least three months' income (and rising), although this is worrying enough, but about his identity being intimately connected to his creative output. Until now I'd underestimated to what extent his sense of self depends on his productivity. His word-count is the yardstick by which he measures himself. The slow erosion of self-esteem brought by not being able to write is adding to his profound sadness at his mother's dying.

As time runs out for Joan, Rory's need to make something of his time is becoming more desperate and – at the same time – less possible. Instead, he is clinging to the minutiae of caring for her, his frustration visible in the dogged intuition with which he's keeping a diary about these days. The notes keep him sane, give his grief a focus and may – one day – help him to make something of this sad experience. For now he has turned this task into a job. I see its necessity, but its nakedness makes me quake at what's to come.

An unsettling side-effect of this is a kind of paralysis on decision making, something he usually finds easy. Now, in even the smallest matters, Rory struggles to be decisive. Of course, in the grand scheme of things it is of no consequence; what does matter is that it is tormenting him and – this is the hardest bit for me – making him hate himself.

I know how essential – and ultimately life enhancing – looking after Joan is; and I am glad that we have been able to offer her a home at the end of her life. I know what is most vital is that Rory and Joan can say goodbye to each other and that we can all treasure this time we have together. But I am afraid of being unable to see into our future, and of imagining that Rory will never be the same again.

Tuesday 14th

Joan: K working. R at his computer. Tess has diarrhoea and wakes us twice in the night. The first finished copy of

Next Exit Magic Kingdom arrives this morning. It has me in stitches. Radio 4 invites R for an interview. R says, 'What the hell am I going to talk about?' *Sunday Times* want to run an extract. M has decided on wedding menu (salmon, Dorset lamb, mixed ices). Sunday's Aussie Grand Prix won by Schumacher in Ferrari. Super start to season with 16 points on Constructors' Trophy. Coulthard and Hakkinen's BMWs both retired with same mechanical problem to their Ilmor-Mercedes engines (pneumatic valve system failure during eleventh and eighteenth laps).

Rory: In a dream I'm driving a VW Camper around a race track. The vehicle breaks down and Mum appears in the stands. She puts aside her Zimmer frame and pushes me to the nearest pit stop.

Wednesday 15th

Rory: 05.45: Mum wakes and pees. I administer five millilitres of Oramorph, help her to her chair, then fall back into bed.

07.15: Our alarm clock rings. Dress. Warm her cranberry juice. Dispense Lansoprazole capsule to protect her stomach. Hang Aid-Call pendant around her neck. She finishes a letter. I walk Tess. Katrin puts on a wash and picks primroses for Mum's bedroom.

08.10: Home carer Pauline arrives. She washes and dresses her. Blue cardigan and silk scarf. Changes her sheets. I refill the birdfeeder. Katrin makes a herbal drink for Mum and toast for herself.

09.10: Katrin leaves for work. I cook oatmeal, mix in honey, fresh mango slices and Maxijul carbohydrate energy supplement. Tub of goat's yoghurt on the side. Carry tray upstairs. Dexamethasone and Thyroxine Sodium. Eat my porridge at computer. Print out Andrew's morning email to Mum.

09.45: Hang out laundry and wash dishes. Mum watches a pair of blue tits. Afterwards, I help her to settle back into her chair, adjust her heating pad, choose another file for her to sort.

10.00: Post arrives. Two letters for Mum from Canada and a form from the council. Water bill for me.

10.20: Social services call to arrange to visit next week. CancerCare Carole confirms her visit this afternoon. Tell Mum, who notes the appointments in her diary. Remind her to put her feet up on the stool to reduce swelling.

10.40: To the post office with Mum's letters. I pay the water bill. In the window is a notice about a lost cockatoo. 'White with scarlet plume. Loud voice. Answers to the name of Jimmy.' Pick up Fruit Pastilles from the shop and next week's drugs from the surgery.

11.15: Make two mugs of tea. Carry them upstairs. 'I'm sick to death of blackcurrant, darling,' Mum tells me. Yesterday she loved blackcurrant.

11.19: Make one mug of peppermint tea.

11.21: Try to write but Mum begins to cough. Help her to find her glasses. Then the top of her felt pen. I sit back down at my desk and stare at a blank screen. I water the plants.

11.55: Book hotel for our weekend in Edinburgh.

12.05: Try to write again.

12.30: Make her lunch: smoked salmon pâté, salad, crackers. Carry tray upstairs. Another Dexamethasone. Aspirin. Grill cheese on toast for me. Eat together.

13.20: Wash dishes.

14.00: CancerCare Carole arrives, neat silver bob and smart suit, discusses labyrinthitis and fear. Next week Mum has an appointment at Dorchester and I don't know how I will get her downstairs and into the car.

'Everything goes woozy,' Mum explains, her voice tightening at the thought of tackling the stairs. 'The steps, the walls, the banisters all start to shake.' She drops her head, ashamed of herself. 'I know it's silly but I can't help it.'

14.35: Carole leaves. Mum is reluctant for her to treat the labyrinthitis, to start another course of drugs. We talk of inconsequential things like fish pie and council tax refunds. We don't mention fear, dying or death. Yet our words have a raw intimacy and we mould the conversation so that it soothes rather than cuts, heals instead of wounds. Then we stop talking altogether and close our eyes.

15.25: Help Mum to the loo. Turn on the tap for her.

15.35: Lay her down for her nap, remembering first to give her the morphine.

15.45: Write diary.

16.15: Wake her with coffee and ice cream. While it melts she walks to the window to watch the birds again. I lift away the frame to hug her.

16.25: Mum picks up Mahfouz's *Palace Walk*. She likes to roll the cool, soft ice cream around her tongue.

17.15: She carries the empty ice-cream bowl to the landing and lays it on the carpet. 'You going exploring, Mum?' I ask.

'I'm just going to walk for a little bit.'

17.25: Finish these notes as Mum coughs in the next room.

18.10: Katrin home from work. She drops shopping bags on the kitchen counter.

I say, 'We're on holiday now.'

'Can you please try to clean up the crumbs after you've cut the bread?' she replies.

18.40: Janet, the evening's home help, deals with evening ablutions.

18.45: Prepare broccoli cheese: onion, olive oil, bay leaf, thyme, coriander, mustard, flour, milk, cheddar.

19.10: Janet leaves.

19.25: Marlie arrives for the weekend.

19.30: Dinner together in Mum's bedroom.

20.45: Wash dishes.

21.00: Katrin calls her friend Christine. Marlie rings Mike. Andrew calls from Toronto. I turn on the television.

22.10: Mum bent over her book, straining both to see and to stay awake. She doesn't want to go to bed early, as she'll then wake us early. Katrin helps her to the bathroom, talks about replanting her penstemon, shares out her cotton pads, dispenses laxatives and morphine.

22.35: Mum swallows a sleeping pill, receives three kisses, lies on her side. Heating pad on. 'Am I lying straight now, darlings?' We place the white stone against her door to keep it from swinging open.

22.50: I take out the dog while Katrin packs a bag.

22.55: Six bedtime biscuits for the dog.

23.25: I'm in bed before Katrin so I can watch her undress. Set the alarm. I open our door six inches wider so I can hear. Switch off the light. Sleep.

Thursday 16th

Joan: Up early as R and K off to Edinburgh by seven. M here for three days, in part to organize reception at Summer Lodge. 'I'm sad whether I'm alone or with you,' she tells me. Afterwards we try on clothes for wedding. Happily, two outfits still fit me. M will lengthen belt of green dress in London. We chat of our travels together: Barcelona, Andalusia, Asia – riding in long boats in Sarawak, her feeling feverish on Tioman Island, waking in beach house to see ships in bay. I discover 1960 diary with her birth – 'a dark-haired daughter' – which makes us both cry. Tendril of baby hair. Sunday she works hard around house: washing sweaters, walking Tess – a lovely girls' weekend. Hopefully, there will be another if R and K go away again. Finish reading Mahfouz's *Palace Walk* – humour, sensitivity to period, character, background of Cairo (Nobel Prize for Literature).

Unfortunately, one of my teeth breaks off.

Saturday 18th

Rory: On the journey north I read Blake Morrison's *And When Did You Last See Your Father?* His chapters have titles like 'Foetal', 'Coffin' and 'Funeral'. He cleaned his father when he soiled himself, heard the last breath, felt the dimming warmth of life in the cadaver hours after death. I find consolation in his experience, but one sentence cuts me to the quick.

'I used to think that solace was the point of art, or part of it; now it's failed the test, it doesn't seem to have much point at all,' he wrote. 'I can't imagine why anyone would want to imagine.'

We're staying in Grassmarket. At lunch, we picnic in the warm sunshine beneath the Castle and gaze northwest towards the Trossachs, impossibly far away. I buy a postcard of a man spreading his arms and flying up into a sky full of birds. At our friends' wedding we dance and talk and drink until I find myself bullying an ambitious, young television producer into having children before it's too late.

Monday 20th

Rory: I've lost patience, sympathy, time. The council miscalculates the refund owed to Mum. I need to write another letter to them. Her final electricity bill is wrong. I need to call. Mum took a mouthful of coffee ice cream and lost an eye tooth. Now I have to find a dentist willing to do a house-call. Irrationally, I blame Marlie for the small tasks left undone. She loves and is loved in equal part. I see how her visits lighten Mum's spirit, that the goal of the wedding – and their joy in discussing it – is keeping her alive. But no matter how much Marlie does – grocery shopping, dropping clothes off at the charity shop, massaging Mum's feet – I feel angry after her departure.

For the weeks after the diagnosis I felt strong. I mourned, steeled myself, prepared for death. There was a perverse solace in the short term. Her – and our – suffering could be contained. It would all be over in eight weeks. Now, with every passing day, I grow weaker and more selfish. My strength to face her illness leeches away. I am less and less able to comfort her pain, to confront the decay of her body. I worry myself sick about not hearing her call, about her swelling stomach, about the car breaking down again.

'I'm falling apart bit by bit,' she tells me.

Tuesday 21st

Rory: For the first time Mum is woken by pain. She gets up, writes a letter, then returns to bed at ten.

'I have a heavy feeling today,' she says.

Her fingers won't let go of her water glass. Last night we cut her steroids from five to four milligrams. Overnight the small reduction has sapped her strength, maybe even given the cancer its head. Four paltry pills are keeping her alive.

'I'll try walking a little,' she says, and shuffles off to watch the birds.

For lunch, Katrin hard-boils a dozen quail's eggs. They were marked down at Tesco. She says they'll make a good wedding-supper starter.

'Do you fancy another nap?' I ask Mum, collecting her tray, expecting her to want to wait until four.

'Yes please. I don't understand why I have so little energy today.'

'I'll wake you in forty minutes,' I tell her.

'Does that suit your plans?' she asks.

'It suits me fine, Mum.'

For supper I fry another mushroom omelette. Katrin is out for the evening.

'I guess it was cutting down on the steroids that made me tired,' she says.

'I think we should go back to the original dose.'

'But I'd like to try to get rid of these,' she adds, rolling up her sleeve. There are black blood blisters on her forearm. 'They're so unsightly.'

Tonight I dream of the theatre. A play ends and the audience applauds as the cast step forward for the curtain call. All the actors are severely disabled. The leading man has no legs, tottering on Dali-esque crutches, a flick of his wrist controlling his forward movement. A young amputee with a backwards foot receives a standing ovation. An elderly actress drags herself across the stage in a wheeled box. I jump to my feet and join in the applause, cheering the crippled performers, willing the show to go on.

Wednesday 22nd

Katrin: Suddenly it's spring. In those first, cold, winter days when Joan seemed to be recovering – blossoming – I loved coming back from work to the tight knot of warmth in our home, bringing with me news, flowers and energy like an aura. Now, in my favourite season, the return of life seems an irony when we are looped about with death. The first warmth of the sun, the smell of freshly cut grass, the urgent twittering of the birds, all gnaw at my heart. I want to shout for joy, to celebrate my love of life, of beauty, of the world to which I belong. But Joan can't come outside and share these simple pleasures, so my heightened feelings turn to a sadness more poignant for Nature's continuity. I think of the tumours growing in Joan's body, like bulbs planted who knows how long ago.

The garden – although a source of such mixed emotions – has become a great solace. We have transplanted most of her plants, integrating them with ours, like the furniture in the house, while Joan – now the vicarious gardener – watches from our bedroom window. Her passion for gardening has become mine, and I prune, weed and re-pot while she nods her approval or gives the 'thumbs-up'. I can now name every plant in our garden thanks to her. My hands in the soil and the action of digging give me the sense that I can create something lasting, while the smell and feel of the earth are like balm to my spirits.

Rory: Late morning Katrin comes inside and says, 'It's so warm in the sun.'

Mum looks down from the window and bites her lip. I can read her regret and say quickly, 'Let's go outside now.'

'Now?' replies Mum, racing to control her fear. 'But . . . but I haven't had any Rescue Remedy today.'

'Right now,' says Katrin, bringing her the Remedy and dripping three drops on to her tongue.

'Up we get,' I say, not giving her time to think, lifting her under the arms.

'It's so beautiful outside,' says Katrin.

We shuffle to the stairs. I'm in front, facing her, walking backwards. Katrin is behind her. 'Put one hand on the banister and the other hand on my shoulder. I'll hold your waist.'

'I don't think I can do it.'

'Of course you can.'

'What if you fall?' Mum asks me, gripping on to the railing, the tendons raised and tense on her bony hands.

'He can't fall,' insists Katrin. 'And I've got you from behind.'

'Come on,' I say.

First step. Second step. Mum whimpers as if she's balanced on a tightrope, or standing in an open aircraft doorway at 30,000 feet.

'Just keep your hand on my shoulder.'

'I can't do it.'

'You *are* doing it.'

'You're doing so well.'

Third step. Fourth step. Turn the corner. Panic. 'I don't know where to put my hand?'

'Just hold on to me. Hold on.'

She wobbles, whimpers again. Fifth step. Sixth step. Her eyes squeeze shut. Her eyes spring open. Her world spins.

'You're doing it, Mum. You're doing it.'

Seventh step. Eighth step.

'Only four more steps, Mum. Three more. Two more. Only one more.'

We are downstairs. Mum grips my hand, and doesn't let go for five minutes. We show her the house plants and pieces of furniture – her furniture – in their new home.

'The prints look good here,' she says.

I lead her out into the garden.

'Now I can see all your hard work, Katrin.'

The sun is hot on our faces. The macrantha is in bud. There's a brimstone butterfly behind the ceanothus.

'The sorbus is late this year.'

We circle the garden. It takes fifteen minutes to walk as many yards. A wren darts into the wisteria. We pick at the pieris and clip the camellia. She says, 'I think I'd like to sit down now, darlings.' She plops into a chair on the lawn, catches her breath, talks about hop compost and an unidentified shrub.

'It's k . . . ke . . . kerria,' she remembers. 'My father called it batchelor's buttons.' Katrin sits on the ground beside her. Tess places a tennis ball at her feet.

'The sun is so lovely.'

I feel like laughing out loud.

Twenty minutes later a thin veil of clouds is drawn across the mild sky. We retreat indoors for lunch. She and Katrin leaf through a gardening book.

'I think we'll have to rethink the position for this one; the book says it grows to five feet.'

I pull labels off pieces of fruit and stick them to her jumper. Cut another sliver of brie. Tell a story. Offer Mum a slice of apple.

'I'd like to go upstairs now,' she answers, 'but I can't remember how to do it.'

The question throws us. She's never before had difficulty going upstairs.

'You usually shoot up,' Katrin assures her.

But she's tired and needs help getting to her feet. We guide her to the stairs, Katrin leading the way.

'Up we go,' I cheer.

'Oh dear,' she quakes.

Twice her legs buckle under her. She grips the handrail with both hands. Her courage falters.

'I can't manage the corner.'

'Just keep going Mum.'

She manages the corner. She makes the last two steps. She pauses, panting, at the top of the stairs. She asks to be helped to bed. I lower the blind. Katrin pulls off her trousers and, as she's hot, her jumper, too. Mum places her hand on her swollen stomach.

'I used to be so flat.'

We lie her down, wrap the heating pad around her waist, pull the duvet over her, close the door behind us.

Later, I join Katrin outside and butcher the euphorbia.

Thursday 23rd

Rory: A wet day. The hills aren't visible through the grey drizzle. The fields are muddy again. A dove ruffles its feathers, perching on a neighbour's television aerial. On the sodden lawn sparrows collect dog hairs to line their nests. I drive Mum to Dorset County Hospital for the appointment she was never expected to keep.

'Is there anything that we can do for you?' Marsden asks her again, a new image of her abdomen in the light box above his head.

We discuss steroids and her lack of appetite. I report on dosage levels and sleeplessness. We're going through the motions. There is no medical reason for us being here.

Marsden proposes doubling her Temazepam.

'Is that wise?' I ask, surprising myself. 'Aren't both Temazepam and Oramorph respiratory suppressants?'

He outlines the options, tries to comfort her.

'I'd like to come and see you again,' requests Mum.

As she's wheeled out of the consultation room, Marsden gestures for me to stay behind. The door hisses shut.

'Are there any questions that you would like to ask?'

I ask about the X-ray.

'The cancer has advanced in both the liver and the lung.'

'In the lung?'

I had thought the lung was clear. He points at the image.

'There's been a change in its contour.'

'And the swelling of her stomach? Is that a tumour?'

'Plus some fluid retention as a side-effect from the steroids.'

'All her life she was proud of her slender figure,' I say.

He purses his lips into a sad smile and tells me, 'She's remarkable.'

'You mean it's remarkable she's still alive.'

On the drive back to the village Mum hides behind her sunglasses. Trees burst into blossom in the fields. Mauve clematis heads peek over roadside roofs. Wessex's old hills roll away to the sea. She says, 'You remember in January that Dr Marsden told you that things might happen suddenly?'

I nod.

'I'd always assumed that he meant quickly.'

I'm lost for words for a moment.

'This . . . change is putting a burden on you and Katrin.'

'You're suggesting that your living on is an inconvenience?'

She smiles. 'It's not what anyone expected.'

'We want you with us at home.'

'I can't get down the stairs alone, which rather puts the kibosh on any plans to run away.'

Five minutes after arriving back at the house, a neighbour rings the doorbell. The radiator of my old Escort has blown out. Yellow coolant streams down the lane. I could fix the leak of course, but having brought us safely back from the hospital, then expired, it seems wrong to demand more of the car. Even machines have their natural span.

Joan: A disrupted night, waking at four – pain on right side so sleeping in quite different way on back with pad at waist. Appointment with Dr Marsden. Some change in liver. Increase sleeping pills. This afternoon CancerCare Carole said, 'He must have been pleased with you.' I asked her about hospice in July when R and K will be in Italy again. She will make enquiries. Tonight R whacked. M has collected wedding shoes, which are fine and comfortable. Mike picked up wedding rings. My left leg dragging.

Friday 24th

Katrin: We hardly need more reminders of the passage of time, but we notched up an anniversary earlier this month: it's now over a year since Rory began taking Chinese herbs to boost our chances of conception.

In last year's diary I marked the number of days between my periods. Over and over again my body deluded me into believing the impossible: thirty-six days, thirty-nine days, thirty-five days . . . To tantalize us, I miss a month, only for a fresh onslaught of emotion (we're awash with it here) when it does, inevitably, arrive. The slow march of time, of hoping without real hope, seems to mirror in miniature our present loss, as Joan's grasp on life slowly slips.

Saturday 25th

Rory: 'Thank you for your Christmas card,' writes Mum. She is forgetting to cross her 't's. 'Unhappily, my health is a bit wobbly and I can no longer live alone.'

As my mechanic takes away the old car, she puts aside her letter to watch the qualifying laps of the Brazilian Grand Prix.

'I didn't know Renault had bought into Benetton,' she says over coffee ice cream.

During commercial breaks she rushes to the loo, not wanting to miss a lap, making herself breathless as if she, too, were travelling at 190 mph.

Joan: K buys strawberries and wicked cappuccino cake, a rival to coffee ice cream. Also a very loving gift of osteospernum for me to see from the bedroom window. She has identified the sweetly scented bush in right-hand bed as winter honeysuckle, *Lonicera*. M phones with news of dress fitting. She says, 'Talking to you has made my day' – as it made mine.

R recounts another dream. He was in a rambling mansion, sorting through papers and possessions: old manuscripts, letters of condolence and rusty dynamos. The telephone rang but he couldn't reach it. A, M and K were blocking his way, sitting in a circle in the hallway, playing cat's cradle. Each strand represented the individual's emotional reaction to my illness. He tried to step over their web, yet it was impossible not to catch the threads and pull on the ties. At last, he managed to find a way through the maze and picked up the phone. But the caller had hung up.

Sunday 26th

Rory: At dawn we're woken by the rooks nesting in the chimney. I stumble up to the attic and throw open the

Velux window to shoo them off. Later in the morning I hang out a Bart Simpson helium balloon to keep them away.

Monday 27th

Rory: Weather turns wintry again, as changeable as Mum's health. Arctic winds gust around the roof, blowing away the balloon. The rooks retreat from the chimney pots to the cover of the trees. Katrin wears gloves on the morning walk. Mum is tired despite a full night's sleep. When I take her hand, I feel her tremble. She swallows two hollow breaths for every sentence. She manages to stomach just half a pear at lunchtime. The Community dentist sticks in her tooth.

'This repair may only last five minutes,' he says.

Later, Mum finishes *Sugar Street*, the last book in Mahfouz's Cairo trilogy. Between chapters she practises walking without her frame, coughing, holding her hands behind her in a 'Prince Philip' posture. She wants to stand straight at the wedding. In the afternoon, when she naps, I update the journal, then read the telephone bill.

'Darling, are you there?' she calls softly from next door.

In the night I dream of walking through a Dickensian Knightsbridge of brooding streets and winding alleys. A worn mesh of metal runs around the edge of a dark square, rusted by time to the iron railings. Outside every house geriatric men and women, alone and in couples, in high Victorian collars and hooped skirts, pick at the rust, peeling away the encrusted past to reveal clean railings underneath. The old residents are putting the square in order, in time for their moving on.

Tuesday 28th

Rory: Mum's tooth falls out while chewing porridge. I put it in a jar of milk in the fridge. On the phone the dentist tells me that a new crown is needed, necessitating two or three visits to the practice.

'A crown will last twenty or thirty years,' he points out, unnecessarily.

Later, our neighbour, Garfield, sprints across from next door, wipes the rain from his glasses and teaches us some tai chi. Mum tries to mirror his graceful movements, her muscles disobeying her, her right hand twisted into a claw.

'Feet shoulder-width apart, knees slightly bent, bum tucked under.'

'I used to be very good at tucking in my bum,' laughs Mum, not acknowledging her jerky actions. When a stretch brings on a cough she says, 'Oh dear, I was breathing in then. What a bad pupil.'

'You need to feel that your feet are grounded,' instructs Garfield, 'and sense the silver thread tying you to the sky and angels. Or whatever.'

Wednesday 29th

Rory: I feel happy, and guilty for it. A telephone call, a small commission and an unexpected cheque make my emotions soar. I bowl into Mum's room, tell her the news, and my enthusiasm almost knocks her over. She closes her eyes against the buffeting.

All day I work on an article, all but forgetting that she is next door. Katrin brings soup for her lunch and cappuccino cake for tea. We take Tess for a longer walk and stop in at a friend's house on the way home. Only after supper do I sit with her. She's moved on from Mahfouz and started reading *Harry Potter*. There are new blood blisters on her hands. The muscles in her arms are wasting away. I tell her about the commission, tempering my zeal, then ask, as I stupidly do every day, 'How are you feeling, Mum?'

'Very well,' she assures me. 'Although I've not been able to use my right hand today.'

I dream that my editor is having a passionate affair with Mum's doctor in a falling elevator.

Thursday 30th

Rory: I am at the cooker when Ruth, a kindly reflex-ologist, rings the bell. It's her first visit and, when Katrin opens the door, I expect them both to go straight up-stairs as the carers do, passing almost unnoticed through my life.

Instead, Ruth steps into the kitchen, sets down her tie-dyed shoulder bag of essential oils and asks me, 'Is there anything I should know before meeting your mother?'

'The cancer is in her brain, liver and lymph system,' I tell her, turning down the cooker. 'Her labyrinthitis, which she managed to control for years, has come back. She no longer has enough courage to fight that, too. Three months ago the doctors gave her eight weeks to live.'

Ruth shivers in the cold rush of fact. 'So we're just trying to keep her comfortable.'

'She's eighty. There is no treatment.'

I meet her eyes. I turn back to the cooker. The months

of living with the disease seemed to have numbed me to its emotional force. I stir the soup.

'I'll take you up now,' says Katrin.

Joan: Ruth is good but too chatty. Next time I will rest my head back and snooze. The treatment is tiring. M rings after final fitting of wedding dress. R and K sorting clothes for car-boot sale. I finish *Harry Potter* – none of the magic or spirit of Narnia but exciting nonetheless. Feeling chilly tonight, even with the heating being cranked up all day, and also a bit blue, despite my success with stairs on Monday.

Friday 31st

Rory: I stick my head around the door frame. 'Ruth will be here in ten minutes, Mum.'

'That reflexologist is no good.' She is rubbing her distended foot. 'The swelling hasn't gone down at all.'

She still believes – or wants to believe – that she will get better, that she's 'getting there', that one day she will walk downstairs unaided.

I ring the dentist to make an appointment for the day before the wedding.

'I'll stick the old tooth back – temporarily,' he says.

In my diary I flick forward through April and shiver. Katrin's friend Christine is due to visit us this Saturday. Marlie and Mike will come next weekend. Katrin's parents are due again on Thursday 13th. We'll clear out the last odds and ends at a car-boot sale while they're here. On

Saturday 22nd Andrew and his family fly from Canada for the wedding. Marlie will be married on Saturday 29th. I close the diary and my eyes. Appointments are made on the assumption of continuity but the only certainty is that continuities end.

Katrin: Joan has always been fastidious over her appearance, increasingly so as her horizons shrink. The lines of her face show her age and her illness, yet still her skin is soft and supple. Though frugal by nature, she once advised me that money spent on quality cosmetics was not wasted. These last three months the small rituals of vanity have been a last bastion of self-esteem against the erosion of her dignity and hope. But this week she has abandoned her daily regime and her moisturizers are untouched on the bathroom shelf.

April

Saturday 1st/Sunday 2nd

Rory: 'I dreamt of your father this afternoon,' says Mum. It's evening now. We're turning in early. 'He was wearing a brown monk's habit which was very unlike him. What do you think it means?'

'That he's here with us?'

'He looked so much younger, like in that photograph. I wish I could remember what on earth happened in the dream.'

'I never dream of him,' I say.

'Probably because he's always off on some adventure,' says Mum.

Four hours later, at about two o'clock, I smell burning toast. Katrin turns in her sleep as if disturbed and at the same instant the lights of two neighbouring houses flick on. Yet outside there isn't a sound.

In the morning I wake to the peal of Sunday church bells and a neighbour's lawnmower. Breaths of cool air sigh through the open window, stirring the blue striped curtains. We listen for Mum and hear nothing.

'I dreamt about death,' Katrin whispers to me.

In her dream, bright sunlight blazed through the high windows of a school assembly hall. Diana, the late Princess of Wales, slipped out of the dazzling light and on to the bench next to her. She handed Katrin four photographs of four little thrones. 'I had them made for my daughters for the wedding.' Katrin and the dead princess took each other's hands. 'You know how things impact on a life,' said Lady Di.

I tell Katrin about smelling burning toast in the night.

'Toast?' she says, turning towards me. 'Do you remember that story you heard about the ghost who announced its arrival with the smell of toast?'

I do. I wrote about it and a spiritualist camp in the Florida book. A psychic there told me that I have a gift to heal. 'Did I tell you that Mum dreamt of my father yesterday?'

'It's like they're all gathering round.'

We realize that we still haven't heard Mum. She didn't go to the toilet in the night. She hasn't slept this late since moving into our house.

Immediately, I imagine that she has died. I run through my memories of the last day: her watch over us as we gardened; her relish tucking into praline cake; her tears of disappointment, sitting alone in the dark for an hour, unable to face the stairs. She had an unexpected call from Canada; the last friend to speak to her. She finished a book by Francine Stock. I remembered the last words that passed between us, me telling her that I love her and she answering, 'I know.'

It would be in character for her to die in her sleep. To cause us as little inconvenience as possible. To take her leave as she has lived her days, with love and care for others. She may even have written us a note, apologizing for the state of the sheets.

I slip out of bed. Had she called out for me in the night and I not heard her? Will I find her hand bell on the floor? Will her eyes be open? Will the body be cold? Will my call catch Marlie before she goes out? Should I wait a few merciful hours to ring Andrew in Canada, to save him from living his nightmare of the midnight call?

I push open the door.

'What a wonderful sleep, darling,' says Mum. 'I've only just woken up.'

Joan: R and K to Castle Gardens to buy hebe and pale lavender. K re-pots the camellia and purple veronica. Garden looks v. frisky. R cuts lawn and afterwards it rains, which will give all the plants a good start. I finish *A Foreign Country* – a first novel about Italians living in Britain at start of war. Good plot. Characterization competent. Structure weak. Late lunch and nap. V. tired tonight – to bed at ten.

Monday 3rd

Rory: It rained all night. Every leaf of every tree is swollen with moisture. I lie in bed listening to the hiss of tyres on wet asphalt. A second balloon has been snatched away by the wind, so the rooks squabble for shelter in our chimney pots again. The laughter of damp schoolchildren rings in the street. As the rain turns to hail and then snow, a winter cloud descends on the West Country. The Mendip transmission tower goes off the air. The Wriggle bursts its banks. Even the dog doesn't want to be outside.

The black cloud also hangs over my day. Mum hasn't died. She is in the room next to my study, awake, breathing, willing to talk until the cough curtails conversation. But instead of asking her about driving an ambulance in the Blitz or if her parents drank wine with supper, I lose my voice. I walk the dog, stand in the field above the village and try to make sense of the last months, grappling to find shape, even prosaic beauty, in the ordinary ebb and flow of hope and despair, denial and acceptance, bloody realism and dreamy fantasy.

Florence Nightingale is also out walking. She hasn't come by the house in a month, thank goodness.

'How's mother?' she asks me.

Everyone else calls her Mum, adopting my name for her as their own.

'The morphine keeps the pain under control,' I say. My lips snap closed like a letter box. I don't want to give anything away, as if withholding intimacies could protect life.

'She's doing *so* well,' babbles Florence.

I'm conscious of my lack of civility. I shouldn't vent my anger at Florence. I force myself to make courteous small talk. But no sooner have I begun than I realize I'm wasting my time. Without another word I turn and run home. The dog can hardly keep up with me. I leap up the stairs, and find Mum too tired even to put a sentence together.

I believe in our ability to shape and direct our lives. I am not fatalistic. But here in my own house, irrespective of the assertions of a Florida mystic, I can do nothing to affect the course of Mum's illness. All I can do is straighten her things while she's out of the room. Her warmth lingers on the armchair. On the floor around it there are illegible Post-it notes and crumpled tissues. I puff the cushions, empty the bin, refill her water glass. I hug her when she shuffles back into the bedroom.

'Can I do anything for you, Mum?' I beg. 'Anything at all?'

Tuesday 4th

Rory: 'I've been very naughty,' she says, eating a white chocolate truffle with her ice cream. 'I haven't sorted any files in weeks.'

She asks me to bring a box of letters from the attic.

'1970s or 80s?' I shout down the stairs.

'Both,' she replies. 'And bring me a big bin bag, too.'

All morning she scythes through a decade's correspondence, pausing only to eat a good lunch: courgette, spinach and broccoli stir fry. Downstairs, Katrin makes preparations for Marlie's pre-wedding dinner, ordering two dozen chicken breasts and two cases of wine. She reserves champagne flutes, books the crockery and arranges to borrow tables and chairs from the church hall. I ring CancerCare Carole from my study to report on Mum's condition. 'She's energetic in the morning, exhausted in the afternoon . . .'

'And practically dead in the evening,' the patient calls from her room.

At six it starts to snow. Denise, this evening's carer, arrives early, worried about being stranded by road closures. Afterwards, Mum complains of pain. I double her morphine and help her to bed, turning on the heating pad. She smiles up at me, red-rimmed eyes and lips the only colour in a white face.

On television a travel show promotes escape to New Zealand. 'Wouldn't you rather be here?' enthuses the presenter.

Joan: 'Whal god is proud
of lhis garden
of dead flowers . . . ?

> . . . lhis body once,
> when il was in bud,
>   opened to love's kisses. These eyes,
> cloudy with rheum,
>   were clear pebbles that love's rivulel
> hurried over . . .
>   . . . I come away
> comforling myself, as I can,
>   lhat lhere is anolher
> garden, all dew and fragrance,
>   and that lhese are the brambles
> about it we are caught in,
>   a sacrifice prepared
> by a lorn god to a love fiercer
>   lhan we can undersland.'

Transcribing R. S. Thomas into my diary while ealing Viennese Whirls. Delicious.

Wednesday 5th

Rory: Katrin tells me that she met a healer at the shop.

'For me?' I ask, hopefully.

'For your Mum,' she answers.

Melanie doesn't make house calls. She prefers to work over the telephone. Katrin rings her for a preliminary discussion.

'Does Joan want to die yet?' asks Melanie.

Katrin answers her questions as best she can by talking about Mum's strength and clarity.

'We have a choice, you know. We can even choose the

date to move on. Then we can have a conscious death, feeling positive, empowered, enriched.'

Mum trusts us and responds positively to Katrin's suggestion that she talk to Melanie. We arrange for her to call in the early evening. Mum sits in the candlelight with the receiver held to her ear. Katrin is downstairs cooking supper. I gravitate between the kitchen and my study, eavesdropping on the conversation:

'I feel loved and cherished so don't understand why I can't throw this thing off,' and 'How on earth can it be my decision?' then finally 'So I'm to acknowledge the cancer's existence?'

After the call we three sit together, holding hands.

'She said that I am responsible for creating the cancer,' worries Mum, her brow knotted and her clarity muddled.

'I don't think she meant it's your fault,' explains Katrin, who spoke to Melanie after their conversation. 'She means that your body made it, so it can unmake it.'

'Oh,' says Mum.

'She believes that you shouldn't fight it.'

'Mum shouldn't fight it?' I repeat, amazed.

'Melanie thinks that if you channel love at the cancer, its destructive power is reduced.'

'"Love your cancer,"' she told me.

'It's a matter of acceptance,' says Katrin. 'It is a part of you, accept it. Love yourself.'

'What bullshit,' I say, regretting our neediness. I'm furious that the vapid pronouncements have confused and distressed Mum. 'I wish we'd never proposed the conversation.'

'She did tell me one useful thing,' Mum says, reaching out to stroke my hand, comforting *me*. 'She saw your father again, Rory, which was lovely. He sent me a message.'

'A message?'

'He told me, "Don't go hurrying along, there's no need for you here yet."'

Thursday 6th

Rory: This morning Mum has no control of her left-hand side. Her head aches and she blames yesterday's reflexology. Katrin cancels the next appointment, telling Ruth, 'The reflexology may or may not have caused the headache but she believes that it did.'

'And she's denying that it may be the cancer,' she replies.

Katrin goes to work. I don't. I make yoghurt, clean the microwave and lie on the floor, disconcerted by Mum's gaze. I don't know if she's taking me in, or simply dazed. She's never suffered from headaches. Now the pain crosses her forehead and wraps itself under her left eye like an evil spirit settling down for a long stay. When I ask her a question, she shakes her head in confusion. When she writes a cheque for the wedding wine, she asks me to help calculate her bank balance. 'Two from six is four, isn't it? And nine minus seven is two.'

I polish another piece of furniture, then bring her coffee. After drinking it, she rallies and asks me to get a new box from the attic.

'Isn't it funny how little work you have at the moment?' she says, as I unpack the files and photographs. 'It's as if we're meant to have this time together.'

We find her diary from the year of my birth ('R sits up in bath by himself . . . listens to his father on the telephone . . . claps his hands') and my adolescent postcards home from summer camp. I uncover my father's briefcase, unopened for thirty years. Inside there's a draft letter from Mum to his lawyer. 'My husband has been very ill and is in hospital. He is recovering slowly from a bronchial infection, but he is weak and we are still on a tight-rope.' One month later he was dead.

'It's good to share this with you,' she says, biting her lip.

Marlie arrives from London with a big Mother's Day bouquet. She has also brought her wedding dress and models it for Mum alone. Downstairs, I make a pot of camomile tea. While it brews I take Tess out into the garden. The night is cool and black. No clouds obscure the canopy of stars. On impulse I go into the garage and begin upending the dozens of rubbish bags. This morning Mum threw out the last picture of my father, snapped in a photo booth. In it he looked broken and sullen, with hair lank and unkempt – it did not portray the man either of us wanted to remember. Now in the papers spread across the grubby concrete floor I find it again, and accept that this is how he looked a few days before he left us forever.

Sunday 9th

Katrin: We had glorious weather for our coastal walk on Saturday. We've come home with the right side of our faces sunburnt from heading east all day. We'd planned to toast the other cheek by walking back the same way today but it was raining hard – and my knees couldn't have managed all those punishing ups and downs again. It felt so regenerative to have a whole day out in the open, striding out, with a single attainable goal – reaching the pub at Worth Matravers before sundown.

I know that, subconsciously at least, Rory has prepared to let go and face death, and understands with acute sadness that he must accept this change. But not knowing *when* he can move on has made him intensely frustrated – a frustration exacerbated by grief. For both of us this has been a therapeutic weekend. It was exactly what we both needed, the best antidote to the last month.

With every step of our walk, the hot sun, the salty wind, the spectacular sea views and the hard, physical effort of climbing, repeatedly, from cliff-top to shore, put distance between us and the illness at home. After the tense, oppressive atmosphere at home, we exulted in physical movement, in breaking away, in seizing the moment.

At Lulworth, where we began, we followed a narrow footpath leading between gorse bushes thick with yellow blossom, and snaked up the cliffs flanking a perfect, clam-shaped cove. Tess ran back and forth, her long pink tongue lolling from her mouth. As we panted upwards, hearts working hard, the shouts of children and the cries of seagulls reached us from the beaches far below. Getting into our stride we could hear, snagged on the breeze, the clear trilling song of skylarks. Their audible relay accompanied us for mile after mile, uplifting and teasing us as we scanned the skies for the tiny spiralling birds that could produce this ethereal sound. Miniature butterflies, coaxed out by the sun, flitted about the gorse and grassland; bees droned drowsily among the plants that flowered atop the cliffs. The sea was a deep Mediterranean turquoise, tempting but icy cold to our hot, tired feet.

We shed layers, applied suncream, paused for breath and snacks, punctuating our eighteen-mile route with stops to bask, to recuperate, to gaze and to marvel. As the sun tilted to the horizon and our limbs grew heavier, our footsteps, breath and energy were all that filled our minds. Even as Joan is dying and no longer able to enjoy these things, we are alive, surrounded by nature whose infinite cycle of death and rebirth is deaf to individual loss, yet is solace to the grieving.

Joan: Glorious sunshine on Saturday. Torrential rain today. M v. sparkly. She and I up chatting both mornings at 6.30 a.m., discussing wedding seating plan. Her dress is magical – a tight, shaped white slip with twin shoulder straps under a beautiful lace gown with long, pointed sleeves – elegant skirt – boat neckline – little train – a wonderful choice. She has also organized flowers: jasmine and freesia in her shower bouquet; bridesmaids to have larger posies, which will double as table centres; lisianthus in window arrangement behind registrar's table.

This morning I tell her it means so much to me that she comes to visit. I also thank Mike for repeating his offer that I live with them but explain I feel settled here. He teasing M about how different things will be after they are married.

'I kind of like them as they are now,' she replies.

Finish Julian Barnes *England, England* – fun and superbly written.

Rory: I ache from the walk. I groan when lowering Mum into bed. 'I'm not sure who's looking after whom this evening,' she says.

Monday 10th

Joan: R keeps stopping me from throwing away papers. He cuts lawn, afterwards wren gathers grass clippings for nest. Creamy yolked quail's eggs for lunch. I suggest to K that in June, when R is away promoting *Next Exit Magic Kingdom*, she invites a friend to stay for walks and chat, so it's not just me here for her to talk to.

Indigestion. Eye inflamed.

Wednesday 12th

Rory: 'I don't know,' she sobs when asked if she wants yoghurt with her fruit. 'I can't make decisions any more.'

I take her hand and tell her, 'Mum, you have cancer. Every day you're fighting it. *Deciding* to fight it. It's no wonder you can't decide about the yoghurt.'

'I just wish I didn't look so awful.'

Three weeks to the wedding.

Thursday 13th

Katrin: Working at Fired Earth three days a week helps keep me sane. The basketry commissions are also a distraction – I've just spent two days on a pair of large log baskets. There's a wonderful rhythm to weaving and I love creating something with my hands and a few basic tools. At the moment I'm even enjoying sorting and soaking the willow – a job I usually hate.

My pottery class, my book club evenings, the occasional massage (gift from Joan), shopping for groceries, swimming, meeting friends for a drink; this ballast helps me function. I need to create the impression of life going on as normal, and in some ways that's all I *am* doing. I cook endless meals – even though Joan only picks at them now – and I go out to work because I see how it helps structure our time.

Friday 14th

Rory: Mum doesn't come downstairs all week. On Tuesday, Katrin went to London to have her hair cut. I can't imagine how a single person manages to care for a dying relative. On Wednesday, she returned with a bell-flowered jasmine plant, filling the bedroom with its honeyed scent.

'But there's nowhere to put it,' I said.

Not an inch of free space remains between the files, photo frames and childhood toys.

'I'll hang it on the walking frame and push it around like a flower barrow,' suggested Mum.

On Thursday, she sat by the sunny landing window, eating a bowl of warmed strawberries, kiwi and banana, smelling the jasmine. Next door in my study with the blind down I did my accounts, and realized I'm running out of money.

This morning Betty, a regular carer, joked, 'You look very rosy today, Mum. Did they have you out in the garden yesterday?'

'They made me do the weeding.'

But CancerCare Carole was concerned. She thinks Mum has become anaemic. Mum asked her again about the hospice. Carole said that she had requested a place. I don't believe her.

'Before then there's the wedding to keep us on our toes,' chirped Mum.

This afternoon Katrin's parents dropped by, delivering a case of champagne for Marlie. They hovered by Mum's chair for a short while, then went away. They said goodbye.

The Times called and asked me to write a humorous article on being a travel writer. 'Can you remember any funny stories?' I ask over supper.

Joan: R has begun to worry that his optimism will be lost with my death. Like me, he has always awoken with a positive attitude. I tell him it's a gift, deeply ingrained, and a part of our nature.

He replies, 'Just to be sure, would you mind sticking around for a while . . . after you've died?'

Sunday 16th

Rory: Another day. One day less. On Saturday it snows again. On Sunday the morning frost steams off the lawn. Both days Mum feels the cold. I turn up the heat, wrapping her in a fleece and a blanket, but she throws them off, determined to keep moving. She orders herself out of the chair. 'Get cracking, Joan.' She's breathless after two steps. I did not believe she could walk any slower.

At lunchtime she has a coughing fit while sipping soup.

The sinews of her neck cord with effort. Marlie's lists of wedding flowers slip like petals on to the floor. I look away, numbing myself, trying not to feel, until I realize that she can't stop the cough.

Is this the end? Should I call an ambulance?

Ninety seconds later she manages to catch her breath. She starts to apologize. I tell her not to speak. A droplet of liquid gathers on the end of her nose. She reaches for a tissue but hasn't the strength to pull it from the box.

'The soup must have gone down the wrong way,' I say.

She shakes her head, her body canted in the chair. There is a stronger brand of morphine, which is to be used only when the fits last longer than *eight* minutes.

'Are you in pain?' I ask her, holding her with both hands. She's not. 'Then we can deal with it.'

She needs to sleep. I lead her to the edge of the bed. I ease off her pale blue jumper and lift her legs. Her feet are like lumps of wax, cool and damp to the touch. As she shrinks towards sleep, I pull the door closed.

I slip downstairs. Tess wants to play. I conjure up a mean game, crouching on the floor, curling my head against my chest and pretending to be dead. The dog runs around me, licking my hands and ankles, nosing my limbs.

After her nap, I sit on her floor. She opens her bloodshot eyes only to reach for her coffee. Her trousers are untidy, her blouse untucked. My fingers can now encircle her thinning forearm. Her bones seem brittle. Again I tell myself to make use of this gift of time, to sit with her, to ask her questions. But she is less and less able to concentrate. Her responses are often dull, lacking her customary wit. She hasn't opened her diary in days. Another fragment of her personality is gone.

'It's so precious talking to you but it's tiring me out,' she whispers. 'I have to conserve my energy.'

We hardly speak for the rest of the weekend. I water her house plants with warm water, as she always did, and empty her wastepaper bin. I help Katrin to clean the house, pulling most of the furniture out of Mum's room to hoover.

'It's so dusty,' obsesses Katrin.

Under her chair I find a file of cards that Katrin wrote to her in the year of our marriage.

'Back then I said how lucky we were to have you join the family,' Mum murmurs to her, holding her hand. 'I want you to know that my feelings haven't changed at all. You are very precious. Take care of yourself.'

Monday 17th

Rory: This morning the house martins return, swooping up under our eaves to reclaim their nests. At the window, I hold Mum for two or more minutes to watch. She drops her head against my chest. Her chin digs into my ribs. I try to imagine that I can feel the organs – both healthy and diseased. I stroke her back slowly.

Warmed fruit and steroids. Salmon pâté and morphine. Asparagus soup with carbohydrate energy powder. Between meals Mum sorts letters. I book a private ambulance to carry her from our house to the wedding and back home. Later in the day, Mary, my BBC producer, calls and asks how long it is until the wedding.

'Twelve days,' I answer.

'She'll make it. But watch her in the days afterwards. Watch her the *night* afterwards.'

Tuesday 18th

Rory: Mum rings Marlie about wedding music. I call the undertaker about funeral music. Katrin's period begins.

Wednesday 19th

Rory: All night it rains. The rivers are flooded again. The road runs alongside a churning stream. On the drive home from the swimming pool I consider steering the car into its frothing, muddy waters.

Katrin shops for the wedding supper: chilli spices, lemongrass and party napkins. She also looks for sandals for Mum. Her feet are so swollen that she will never fit into her dress shoes, even with their sides cut.

In the evening I can't pull myself away from *ER*. As Katrin does the ironing, dispenses drugs and tucks Mum into bed, I escape into a medical drama double bill.

'More suction, damn it.'

'BP 132 over 82.'

'Watch the pancreas; the bastard really sliced the hell out of it.'

I used to watch television rarely, now I turn it on every night. On screen, a deranged patient knifes two doctors, an old lady passes away and two children are orphaned by a car accident.

'Lucy's dead, isn't she?'

I find myself crying over an actress in a TV soap.

'Call it.'

'Time of death: 03.26.'

Thursday 20th

Rory: Wind and rain then an hour's searing sunshine. Dandelions lift yellow heads to mock my gardening skills. Mum had a bad night and, as she shuffles to the bird window, makes shallow animal grunts. Between breaks in the clouds we see two greenfinches and the wren.

'Is there a crematorium near here?' she asks me quietly. I've been waiting for months for the question. 'It's something that we should talk about.'

'Yes, Mum. There is one nearby.'

'I don't think I want much of a funeral.'

'Just the family?'

'Just the family.'

She asks me to remind her about her brother's funeral. She's forgotten the details. I tell her it was a simple affair with a minister who didn't know him.

'I don't want our village vicar. He refused to marry Marlie simply because Mike is divorced. Pray for forgiveness on Sunday then refuse to marry two people in love on Monday; that's hypocritical. I don't want him there.'

'I've been trying to imagine the service – Andrew reading a prayer, me reciting a poem, Marlie probably too moved to speak – and then you're . . . gone. It feels so lonely.'

'Without me?'

'Without you. Also without someone to hold it – and us – together.'

'But we only know the local man.'

'Every morning when Katrin and I walk Tess we meet a retired, bearded minister coming back from the shop.'

'I've seen him.'

'He always has a kind word, or makes a joke. He likes that Katrin and I hold hands, and that I fly a balloon from the roof to scare off the rooks.'

'I like the sound of him.'

'I don't know his name but he's a Scot. He may be a Methodist.'

'It doesn't matter what he is.'

'I could ask him if he'd be willing to conduct the service, just to give us a . . . framework.'

'Do you think – when I get less strong – that he might come and see me?'

'I'm sure that he would. Then he'd have met you and – afterwards – every morning when we pass him he would be a link back to you.'

Friday 21st – Good Friday

Rory: Katrin is home all day so I work, sketching out *The Times* article. Over lunch I ask Mum to read the first draft. I want her to remain involved and to keep her busy. I'm also accustomed to listening to her advice. But when I collect her lunch tray she hasn't understood the piece. I thank her and smile but as I carry the remains of the meal downstairs I want to throw the tray on the floor and crush the bottles of pills.

Later, she asks me about the subject of my next book. Healing in California? Retracing the hippie trail? A first novel? I tell her that in time I'd like to write about these days together.

'You don't mind me writing about you, Mum?'

'As long as it's not too syrupy. I know whatever you write it will be done with sensitivity.'

Saturday 22nd/Sunday 23rd – Easter weekend

Rory: Andrew, his wife Margaret and son Neal fly from Toronto to London. They're spending three days in town before coming to Dorset.

Mum watches the qualifying laps of the British Grand Prix at Silverstone. She regrets missing the San Marino round. Her friend Maggie from Wimbledon visits for the night, bringing books and sitting with her while we prepare roast lamb. We eat it together on the landing. Over the meal my speech is muddled, even before the first glass of wine. These days I often slur my words and drop syllables. 'Will you have one or twee potatoes?' 'Red or white vin?' I'm becoming forgetful, too.

Sunday morning Katrin and I escape from the scream of Formula One tyres to plan the year ahead: *Next Exit*'s launch in June, Italy in July, the Edinburgh Book Festival in August, then maybe California. We reach out from a Wessex woodland towards the Pacific.

Back home, after qualifying rounds and croissants, Maggie reports that Mum asked if she is a burden on us.

'I don't want to damage their marriage,' she told her, then cried.

While David Coulthard wins the Grand Prix, Mum writes the dates of my reading tour in her diary. She asks Katrin to buy her extra shampoo, even though there are two full bottles in the cupboard. I will her to live on, and feel my heart sink. I want it to end, but then I'll never see her again.

Katrin: There's so much to do before Marlie's big day. I've thrown myself into arranging the pre-wedding dinner. I love imagining every last detail, though I wish sharing it could be a little more fun.

Still, I'm enjoying devising the menu, buying ingredients, organizing the seating and decoration of the living room, deciding which rugs to put where. I've bought fabric to drape over the dresser where we'll serve the drinks, and Chinese paper, painted with small squares of gold and orange for luck, to scatter beside the glasses. I've renovated terracotta saucers for cayenne and celery salt to go with the quail's eggs; they'll be served in baskets along with an assortment of different breads. I've re-potted plants from the market and decorated them with coloured ribbons, and printed card place settings with 'm & m' – Marlie and Mike – like the sweets of that name . . .

Having Maggie to visit brought us together again. Though I've become a poor judge of time, it felt like ages since we last sat and talked and shared a meal together. When Rory drove her to the station, I sat with Joan and showed her the dainty saxifrage for the tables in their pretty pots. It was so precious to be alone with her again. I realized that, unconsciously, I'd been avoiding her because I couldn't face the idea that she would soon be gone. With the house about to fill up for the wedding, this was my last chance to share this fear – and to tell her how much I loved her. There are few people with whom I could imagine having such a conversation, but with Joan it felt the most natural thing in the world. I told her that her courage and convictions have built a bridge for me into the next world.

Tuesday 25th

Rory: Our eighth anniversary. Eight years to the day Andrew, Margaret and Neal return here, importing laughter and half a dozen suitcases into the house.

Andrew embraces Mum, then retreats to the threshold of her bedroom door, shocked by her appearance. Margaret barrels past him, kneels on the floor and says, 'Oh Mum.' Katrin has prepared their lunch and supper. The drugs are laid out on my desk. I've even rigged up an old battery-powered bicycle siren and placed it beside her bed. It will wake even the deepest sleeper. I'm treating Katrin to a surprise trip to London. She and I drive away, spending the afternoon tripping between Tate Modern, a Thameside walk, cocktails and a Japanese dinner in Soho. We fall asleep on a sofa bed in Acton, a thousand miles away from home. Katrin wakes without a neck ache for the first time in two months. We return home by way of Ikea, buying a new light fixture for the shower room and three hundred candles.

Wednesday 26th

Joan: R and K in London. A, Margaret & Neal are v. dear and helpful. A pleased with progress of his new company – outlined various developments he wants to explore – sees a good future. Margaret, as expected, is wildly excited about the wedding. She's v. taken with Mike. Gives me a good twenty-minute leg massage to reduce swelling, which eases walking.

Reading Agatha Christie's absorbing autobiography – all her own unusual life, broken and happy marriages, story of path to success.

Delirious.

Thursday 27th

Rory: The dentist is booked for this morning but Mum can't face the stairs.

'I don't want this toothy grin to ruin the photographs.'

I assure her that the gap is only visible in a broad smile. I also remind her that the repair would be temporary.

'You mean if I make the effort today, the tooth may fall out tomorrow?'

I tell her that it might, just as I told her a month ago.

'The long-term solution is to make a new crown,' I say.

On our morning walk, Katrin and I run into the retired minister. I explain the situation and ask him if he might be able, and willing, to guide us through the funeral service.

'Afterwards we'll be able to see you every day and you are of this place.' I bend down and tap the tarmac with my knuckles.

'I'd be honoured to be of service,' he replies with a Lanarkshire lilt, agreeing to drop by early next week after the wedding. Then he takes our hands.

Back at home, Andrew lies on the bed talking to Mum. I join them to recount our talk with the minister, saying out loud the words 'funeral' and 'cremation'.

'We were just talking about my popping off,' Mum tells me.

An hour later I'm loading the fridge with bottles of champagne when the doorbell rings. It's the minister.

'I thought why wait until next week? If it's convenient, I could meet your mother now.'

Mum is upstairs, writing out the wedding-supper place cards.

'I hear you're going through the wars, lass,' he says, and asks her about Canada. 'How long did you live there?'

'Over forty years. I married a Scot.'

'Oh dear, no,' he laughs.

'Then I moved back to England.'

'I came to England myself . . . as a missionary.'

'Have you had much success?'

'Very little.'

He asks if he could give her a blessing, takes her hand and prays.

I still don't know his name. At the front door he gives me his card. An address label stuck on to a snip of cardboard reads John McMinn.

'I made them myself.'

Outside a light breeze stirs the pink heads of the clematis above the back door. Newborn chicks cheep in the wisteria. Tess rolls on her back and sniffs the spring air as sparrows snatch more clumps of moulting hair to line their nests. I collect the chicken for tomorrow's supper and borrow a wheelchair from the surgery. Andrew collects the tables and chairs from the church hall. Our neighbour, Garfield, helps us unload the car.

'Your mother's dying and you're having how many for supper tomorrow night?' he asks.

'Twenty-five.'

'But . . . why?'

'To celebrate life.'

Come 10 p.m. Marlie has arrived from London. I open the first bottle of Lanson and she calls this her hen night. While Margaret tries different make-up combinations on her, she chats to a friend in Australia.

'Obviously, Mummy's illness isn't that good, but it's so great that she's here.'

In the kitchen, Katrin is cooking three enormous pots of Thai chicken. In my study, Andrew and I refine our speeches. Next door Mum is coughing – the morphine is ineffective this evening – and writing up her diary again.

Thirty-six hours to go.

Joan: Cancelled dentist to conserve strength. John McMinn dropped by at R's request – a devout man – R and I both liked him – sincere and moving blessing touch for R and me – I feel happy that he will set a framework for my cremation. Neal transfixed by television snooker. M arrived full of hugs – good drive down from London. We opened champagne and drank to her; the last time we are all MacLeans.

Friday 28th

Rory: I drive into Sherborne three times to run errands and collect forgotten items: fresh coriander, mangoes, raspberries, whipping cream – and morphine. Marlie bubbles and laughs while arranging the flowers. Margaret massages Mum's feet with peppermint oil as Andrew lays the tables in the living room. We've rented linen, cutlery and china. There are flower pots and floating candles, celery salt and place names. Katrin arranges bowls of pebbles in water, stirs the curry, hoovers the hallway.

The evening's carer helps Mum into a long mauve dress. Marlie finds the pearls. We manage to squeeze an adjustable pair of sandals on to her feet. Ten minutes before the guests arrive Andrew and I steer her to the stairs.

'Oh God,' she says, again and again, grabbing for the banister.

Her chair awaits her at the bottom of the stairs. We guide her to it, sit her down. Marlie finds a missing earring.

The guests – Mike's relatives, Marlie's new family – arrive and Mum stands to shake their hands. Andrew's arm is around her waist. I pop corks. We toast the couple, talk, refill our glasses.

'Such a beautiful house in a secret little village . . .'

'On the Upper East Side behind the Guggenheim . . .'

'You must stay with us in Brussels . . .'

We sit down to eat in the living room, happily bumping elbows and voices. Mike's grandmother, Magda, is twelve years older than Mum, a bird-thin, robust nonagenarian who loves spicy food.

'Ten years I have lived away from Europe,' she tells Katrin in a thick Hungarian accent. 'Ten years I've tasted nothing this strong. It is wonderful.'

Mum's fingers shake as she shells the eggs. Her place setting is showered with their fragments, as if someone had been grinding them into the tablecloth. I lay three rolls of salmon on her plate. She eats only an edge of chicken, talking energetically to Mike's daughter by his first marriage: medical school, boyfriends, a working holiday in India.

Mum needs to go to bed before dessert. Andrew and I lead her upstairs. Marlie helps her undress.

'You've done so well,' we tell her, kneeling together beside her bed.

'At least we've kept up the subterfuge.'

When we return to the party, Mike's father says to me, 'I do not know much about illness but your mother does not look like a woman who is letting go of life.'

Joan: K's organization was superb – everything flowed according to plan: devilishly spicy curry, crisp vegetables, exotic fruit salad. Mike's father, Edmond, wonderfully polished and diplomatic. He told A, 'Your mother has done well bringing up children on her own . . . deserves great credit for such a fine family.' His mother, Vera, most vibrant. Host of enchanting children. Champagne toasts to M and Mike. M taking great care of me.

Katrin: What a strange evening. I spent half of it meeting new people, the other half waiting for Joan to pee.

Saturday 29th

Rory: Wedding day. Marlie calls my name at five o'clock. The dawn is thick with mist and birdsong.

'I haven't slept all night,' she says. 'May I have a sleeping pill?'

'But they last for six hours.'

'If I don't have one, I'll be so tired . . . and look awful.'

Two hours later Mum rings her bell. She's sitting on the edge of the bed in the sunshine. 'I've got no energy this morning.'

'Mum, it's early. I haven't got any energy yet either.'

'But I can't even stand.'

I help her to her feet and calm her anxiety by recounting her success last night.

'We made a good performance,' she says, a contented smile curving her pale lips.

I offer to bring her a warm drink.

'And some fruit salad, please. I missed it last night.'

I increase her steroids for the day.

The morning sky is cloudless. Marlie sleeps, wakes and assembles her dress, suitcase and overnight bag together in the front hall. She and Katrin adjust flowers and debate lipstick colour. She sits alone with Mum, then with Katrin and Margaret drives to Evershot, the village where the wedding is to take place.

An hour later, Di, today's carer, arrives, dressing Mum in the green dress that she wore to both my and my brother's weddings. I'm cast in the role of wardrobe assistant. I can't find her petticoat. The belt no longer fits around her waist. I pick off the poppers and fasten it with a safety pin. The straps of the sandals dig into her swollen feet.

'Don't forget my pearls. Where are my earrings?'

She doesn't lie down for a late-morning rest. For lunch she drinks only a mug of soup. Neal grills himself leftover Thai chicken on toast with cheese and ketchup.

The ambulance arrives five minutes early and Mum is still on the loo. 'Bother,' she swears.

The crew carry her downstairs, her dress billowing over the carry-chair. We drive in convoy to Summer Lodge and wheel her into the hotel library.

Marlie enters wearing an elegant silk dress under a flared skin of Flemish lace. There are freesias in her hair. She looks beautiful. In my pocket are confetti and Fruit Pastilles.

The simple civil ceremony is moving and sincere, witnessed by thirty-five family and friends. Andrew and I sit on either side of Mum, helping her to stand and sit, guiding her to Marlie afterwards. She whispers while kissing her, 'Darling, darling Marlie.' The euphoria – and the steroids – lift her strength, increasing her animation and carrying her along. She wants to walk unaided to the garden for champagne but the queue bunches up behind her in the corridor so we whisk her back into the wheelchair and out into the sun.

'I don't want the chair in the photographs,' she gestures and Andrew spirits it away.

Mum sips champagne, kisses new relatives, forgets about her missing tooth. Her broad, gappy smile is caught in a hundred photographs. She looks both radiant and tired and needs to lie down for half an hour before the meal.

'All my life I do ten minutes' exercise every morning. That is my secret for longevity,' Mike's grandmother tells me.

At the table I sit beside her and across from Mum. A bridesmaid's bouquet is at the centre of each of the four tables. Mum eats her salmon starter but hardly touches the lamb.

'These are beautifully written,' says Magda, picking up a place card. She's been briefed.

'Our Mum wrote them,' adds Andrew.

'Such elegant handwriting.'

French waiters from Yeovil sweep away plates and pour more wine. We time the speeches for before dessert. Andrew and I speak in a double act, first about Marlie's difficult childhood – that is, growing up with two elder brothers – then, as she matured, our difficulty in coming to terms with her beating us at tennis, squash and school. We propose a toast to her and absent family.

After the speeches, Mum tells Andrew that she's ready to leave the party. He alerts the ambulance crew but she changes her mind. The cake is still to be cut. As we wait for a knife and plates, she worries that she hasn't spoken to all the guests. When coffee is poured, she tries to get to her feet. 'I think I'd better go home now, darlings.' Andrew and I steer her to the door. Her chair is secreted in a side passage. We wheel her to the ambulance. Katrin climbs in beside her. Marlie and Mike bring cake and chocolate for the crew. Mum lays her head back on the stretcher and closes her eyes. The newlyweds wave off the bride's mother.

Joan: M looked v. elegant, beautiful and rather Spanish with flowers in back of hair – her bouquet an exquisite arrangement of delphinium, verbena and monkshood interwoven with ivy and olive green ribbon. Her and Mike's pledges to one another were touching – 'I want to spend my life with you' – bridesmaids' dresses pretty – whole setting attractive. Sorbet delicious – lamb disappointing to me. Speeches by R and A v. funny and most people thought spontaneous. R said, 'There is one other person who, though not involved in choosing Marlie's dress, was intimately involved in creating the package it's wrapped around. That's our father, who would be so proud of her if he were here today – and maybe he is.' Much applause. Spirit of love in the room. I left in ambulance, I think discreetly.

Sunday 30th

Rory: The night is mild and clear. Andrew sleeps in the attic room with the Velux window open, watching the stars.

On Sunday morning, Mum calls us into her bedroom.

'Look what just fell out,' she says. In her palm is a gold crown. 'I'm getting quite a collection.'

'Lucky we didn't bother with the dentist.'

'Perhaps we should melt it down and make some money.'

'To buy more coffee ice cream,' suggests Katrin.

We clean the house, strip the beds, breakfast on a new stash of chocolates brought by Vera and Edmond from Brussels. The wine glasses are returned to the off-licence. The furniture is restored to its usual place. Katrin does three washes. Margaret massages Mum's feet again. Five times she asks Andrew, 'When are you leaving, darling?'

'Three o'clock, Mum.'

She sits in her chair, turning the reading lamp on and off. On and off. Last night, while removing her make-up, she couldn't stop patting her face with the cotton pad.

Marlie and Mike stop by for an hour *en route* to Heathrow, glowing with happiness. It's possible that Mum may not be alive when they return from honeymoon.

'Don't think about anything here,' I tell them.

'We'll call you from Morocco,' says Marlie.

'No we won't,' says Mike with a wink.

Andrew and Margaret pack. Neal organizes his school books. I melt cheese on a toasted bagel for Andrew's lunch, bringing it to him and Mum in her room. The rest of us eat in the kitchen. I load their suitcases into the car. Just before three Andrew and Margaret are saying goodbye to Mum, talking about flight times and remedies for snoring, inconsequential topics that won't enflame the last minutes, when the doorbell rings.

'I thought I'd drop by and see how you got on yesterday,' says John the minister.

Margaret – who is a devout Christian – takes his hands. 'You are the answer to our prayers.'

At three o'clock Andrew bows forward into an unnatural stoop and embraces Mum. She tries to put her arms around him but only manages to reach his waist. He holds her frail, bent frame for the last time. His eyes are shrunken and red. Her fingers are shaking. I look away. Katrin goes downstairs into the shower room to cry.

Then they're gone.

May

Monday 1st

Katrin: Suddenly it's May, my birth-month, my best time of year. Yesterday I heard the first cuckoo but my elation was short-lived – I am haunted by the image of Andrew holding Joan in his arms for the last time. It seemed so abrupt to leave each other that way; a clumsy embrace to conclude a lifetime's love, a full stop, which ends this part of their story. Then to drive away, knowing they would never see each other again. How could Andrew bear the pain of saying goodbye? Surely his heart must have burst into a thousand tiny pieces.

Now the house feels so quiet. It's a bit like New Year after the excitement of Christmas – a note of realism but without the new beginning. We've retreated into our own corners, tired and a little unable to look each other in the eye.

We were bound to feel a sense of anti-climax after the wedding but it's also a huge relief to have it behind us. As stressful as the build-up has been, there were, of course, many wonderful moments to the weekend. Saturday was such a glorious sunny day and Summer Lodge a beautiful, well-chosen setting. An old brick wall shelters the large garden, so we were outside for drinks and photos. A magnolia tree was covered in blossom and, to one side, under the shade of tall beech trees, delicate fritillaries – one of Joan's favourite flowers – nodded among the moss. Marlie, Margaret and I, sisters-in-law together, got dressed in a suite of elegant rooms at the hotel, putting on our make-up and laughing over well-chilled English wine. Bride and groom were deliriously happy.

And Joan made it through most of the day, though as time progressed I became more conscious of the filminess of her skin, its texture and puffiness, each shadow a sign of her illness. Most of the day I was waiting for the signal that she was ready to go home. It was odd to be at a wedding where my attention was not focused on the bride and groom.

I'm glad to have the house to ourselves, but I already miss Andrew and Margaret's support and energy. We're pared down to our essentials now, treading water. Waiting and tiring.

Tuesday 2nd

Rory: A limbo descends on the house. The clock on my desk has read nine for hours. Katrin is downstairs trying to read Beryl Bainbridge's novel on the Titanic. I've just jerked myself awake from a dream of flood waters rising around a tumbledown cottage. I tried to plug the gaps around an ill-fitting door, ignoring the gleaming modern aircraft waiting on the hill behind that could spirit me away to safety. Next door Mum is dozing over a novel about Henry VIII, crumpled in on herself, shrinking into her body.

Yesterday Katrin ran in from the garden, excited, calling up to us, 'Do you hear the cuckoo?' An hour later her happiness had evaporated. 'So what happens now?' she whispered, as if speaking out loud might tear us all apart.

For four months Mum has beaten the cancer, answering visitors' enquiries with, 'Quite well today, thank you.' I wonder if now I should help her to find a new goal. But I don't want to sugar her with false optimism. Her diary is filled with dates yet there is no single, poignant event on the horizon for her to live for. Only her will could extend this period of grace.

Her physical condition has changed dramatically these last weeks. 'I think I'll have a walk now' used to mean half an hour motoring back and forth between the bedrooms. Now it's an exhausted, snail crawl to the loo. Her swollen liver presses on her diaphragm, making her breathless. It's squashing both her stomach, killing her appetite, and her bladder, giving her the sensation of needing to urinate. Bladder dysfunction predisposes her to urinary infection, which could cause confusion and delirium.

Our conversations are different, too. A month ago I'd lie on her floor for two or three hours at a time, reflecting and speculating. By contrast the silence has almost embarrassed us these last days. We've said little of value. My little jokes – the day-to-day teases – no longer engage her. She takes them literally, nodding with eyes closed, then tips far to the left in her chair and falls asleep.

Two visitors come by today. CancerCare Carole arrives first. Before he returned to Canada, Mum asked Andrew to list the changes in her since his last visit. 'What the hell can I write?' he had whispered to me. This afternoon Mum reads his list aloud to Carole.

'Less mobile. Less energy. Swelling legs . . .'

I suggest that she also mentions the wiggly lines that now dance before her eyes.

'I just read for too long yesterday.'

Instead of the usual twenty minutes, Carole stays for over an hour, sitting by the bed, feeling Mum's stomach, stroking her legs. Afterwards at the front door she says to me, 'It's magic wand time.'

I remember reading of an American oncologist's advice to his patients: hope for the best, prepare for the worst and pray for a miracle.

'Do you have a wand?' I ask Carole.

'It's the one thing they didn't give me.'

Later, a doctor from the Dorchester hospice stops in at Mum's request. She intends going there in July so we can have our summer holiday, which we will cancel of course if she's still alive ('By the way, Mum, if you die now, we can go on vacation'). The doctor examines her, discusses her breathlessness and takes her one step closer to the unknown.

'Are you feeling any pain?'

'No,' she answers. 'Not at the moment.'

'Mum had a lot of abdominal pain last month,' I volunteered, pushing them both to be more candid.

'And what do you think caused it?' he asks her.

'The coughing,' she responds. 'If only I could stop coughing.'

'Do you think it could be something to do with your illness?'

Pause.

'Of course.'

At the front door again, where truths are spoken openly, he tells me, 'It's optimistic to think that she will live until July.'

'Is there any medical reason for her to go into a hospice?'

He shakes his head. 'There is nothing we could do that you aren't doing here.'

'Since we have to lose her, let it be in a place she knows and where she's loved.'

An hour later, while Katrin is massaging her feet, Mum

says to her, 'My resolve is strong while I'm here. I feel safe in this house. But if I had to go to a hospital, I'm not sure that my resolve . . .'

Her words falter and she cries. Tears roll down her cheeks and fall on her bulky, dishevelled sweater. She tucks the fleece around her. She whispers, 'I'm not getting better.'

Wednesday 3rd

Joan: Awake at 4.50. Dressed and in chair by 5.15. Sunny at six. Left leg sore, painful. Luckily, acting district nurse Jane is on duty – demonstrated foot/leg exercises to reduce swelling. Marked improvement. R writes short article on Florida mermaids for Virgin Atlantic in-flight magazine. All tired – reaction to M and Mike's wedding. Flowers still looking exquisite, especially M's bouquet. One blue tit on feeder.

Rory: 'Can you bend your foot at the ankle, my sweet?' asks Jane. She's round, caring and smells of menthol cigarettes. 'That's it. That's brilliant.'

'I'm glad I'm brilliant.'

Mum is losing co-ordination and orientation. Her leg sores are weeping. Her swollen feet look like tubers and she can no longer move them backwards. I find it more and more difficult to guide her on to the toilet, to turn, to reach back and to lower her on to the seat. 'Am I there now? Am I squared up?' She knocks her hip against the arm of the commode. She's fretful about wetting herself so sits on the loo for half an hour five or six times a day. Three hours a day. When she stands, I adjust her clothes and see broad, red marks on her thighs.

'I'm so useless.'

'What on earth are you talking about?'

'I can't do anything. Could you help me pull down my trousers, please?'

'But I've just helped you to pull them up.'

She's out of breath and she doesn't want to lose the urge. She sits down on the seat, almost missing it.

'I'll leave you five minutes, Mum.'

'I may be longer.'

'Ten minutes then.'

'I don't want to disturb you.'

'Don't worry. So five or ten minutes?'

'Five or ten?' She shakes her head. 'Whatever you want.'

Pears and apricot compote for breakfast, warmed in the microwave to release the flavour. The way she likes them. Strawberry yoghurt to help ease down her pills. She coughs all morning.

Katrin measures out the morphine, brings up a tray at meal times then afterwards carries it back downstairs, the food never more than half eaten. This afternoon she books herself a massage. Mum takes some notes from her purse and squeezes them into her hand. 'My treat.' She tries to read *The Vintner's Luck*, her left hand holding the book, her right finger tracing the lines of text. I doze on her floor. Around two o'clock a train passes through the village's request-stop station.

'I love the sound of the trains,' she says. 'I hear the whistle and wonder if anyone will be waving their umbrella.'

For supper I bring her a few rolls of smoked salmon. She slices them into small pieces and chews them slowly with her mouth closed. She and Di, the evening's carer, are in the bathroom when Marlie calls from Ouarzazate.

'It's taken us an hour to get through,' she shouts. 'Please can I speak to her?'

I lean around the door. Mum is braced against the sink as Di soaps her bottom. I hold the receiver to her ear.

'Hello, darling. Everything's fine here. You've been through the Atlas Mountains today? How lovely. Have a wonderful honeymoon.'

Di keeps washing throughout the conversation. 'It's a good thing you don't have one of those picture phones,' she says afterwards.

Later, Katrin and I sit downstairs watching *Out of Africa*. When we put her to bed, Mum says, 'It was lovely to hear the music.'

Thursday 4th

Rory: 'Unfortunately, the pain has come back on my right-hand side.'

It's five o'clock in the morning. Mum sits on the edge of her bed, one foot jammed under Lightning. She doesn't want to walk to the bathroom. Carole's suggestion that she 'conserve her energy' has changed her attitude. Suddenly she's being easier on herself.

I wheel her to the bathroom and go back to bed. Thirty minutes later she rings her hand bell.

'Do you want to walk back to your room?' I ask her.

She shakes her head. I push her across the hall, then shuffle and roll her back into bed. I lay the heating pad over her ballooning belly, administer her Oramorph, spilling a few drops, then turn off the light.

When I get up at seven, she's sitting on the edge of the bed again. 'It's still hurting,' she says, holding her side.

'I spilt a lot of the Oramorph,' I lie, giving her another dose.

I help her into the chair and bring hot cranberry juice. She starts a thank you note to Marlie and Mike. 'Il was such a lovely surprise to have your call lasl nighl . . .'

At nine, Betty, this morning's home help, rings the bell.

'How's Mum?' she asks at the door. Usually Betty storms in, greets the dog, drops her bag and thunders upstairs. This morning she hovers at the foot of the stairs.

'She's slipping, Betty,' I say.

'I heard yesterday that she wasn't so well.'

No energy for hair washing today. After dressing her, Betty props Mum up in bed to try to drain her feet.

'Is it chilly in here?' Mum asks. 'I feel quite cold.'

The thermostat is set at 75°.

The morning is overcast. Above the low, dull clouds the sun must be blazing. It will be hot in Morocco. With my window open, I try to do a little work. A travel editor isn't returning my calls. I worry that I'll never again leave the house. I write my book-festival talk.

Mum calls me in to help her make another decision. 'Darling, should I sleep now or have lunch?'

'Are you hungry?'

'Not at all.'

While she dozes, John the minister rings the bell. In his hand he holds a potted plant. I turn him away. 'Please come back tomorrow,' I tell him.

'I will. Bless you.'

Joan: Cold, grey morning. Sunshine at noon. Jane checks legs – pleased with progress. John brought blue lisianthus – couldn't find the moment to ask him the personal questions on faith as I had planned. Finish *The Vintner's*

Luck – Burgundy 1808: one night Sobran Jodeau, a young vintner, meets an angel in his vineyard, a gorgeous creature with huge wings that smell of snow. A strange and moving book that touches the heart on the struggle for souls between God and Satan.

Rory: At five o'clock, after her nap, Mum finally urinates; the first time in twenty hours. I wheel her back to her room and help her towards the armchair.

'Which way do I go? Right or left?'

'Right, Mum. Your chair is here beside you.'

She slumps into her seat, winded. 'I feel like I've just crossed the Arctic.'

I bring her a late lunch of salad and a few more slivers of smoked salmon. She asks for more morphine.

'It's a nuisance that this pain has come back.'

With my mug of tea I sit on the floor, hoping to talk. She asks me about the day's writing, then closes her eyes. I wait. I close my eyes, too. We doze in silence. Sometime later she reopens her eyes. 'I can't figure out when I lost my faith in God,' she says.

'Maybe after Dad died,' I reply. 'Although you went to church every Sunday for the following year.'

'I must have believed then. Or at least still had a child's view of God sitting on his throne in Heaven, answering our prayers. I was taught that all one had to do was call. But He didn't come to help me.'

'I think He did, in a way.'

'He didn't bring your father back.'

'But his death brought us closer together. We were our own community.'

We fight and resist loss throughout our lives, knowing all along that life cannot change without it. I turn out the light. Mum sits in the dark, her arms stretched above her head, heating pad strapped to her waist, confronting anew her aches and fears.

Friday 5th

Rory: Suddenly Mum isn't walking. Her only independent movement is the bed-to-chair shuffle, which she does while clinging to me. I wheel her back and forth to the bathroom on Lightning. She ventures no farther. She eats a few spoonfuls of fruit salad and the indigestion returns. We discover that soda water helps to settle her stomach.

Boxes go unsorted and calls unanswered today. Weeds sprout in the garden. In the afternoon, Jane calls by again to check on her feet. She notices the uneaten meals.

'I hardly touched my breakfast or lunch,' confesses Mum. 'Can you give me something to settle my tummy?'

Jane is worried about malnutrition.

In the evening, John the minister tells us that he has lost his cat. 'I think that I'll have to let it be part of the past,' he says.

Saturday 6th

Rory: The weatherman predicts storms. Like a horticultural chemotherapist, I spread weed killer on the lawn and wait for rain. But the sun burns through the clouds and the day turns hot. I now can't let Tess outside on to the lawn.

The birds desert the garden. The whole house stinks of chemicals.

Katrin goes to work, taking the dress Mum wore to Marlie's wedding. She will never wear it again but she wants it dry-cleaned. Over lunch – or at least over the uneaten bowl of breakfast oatmeal – she talks about the theatre.

'Before the war I tried for the Old Vic.'

Her audition piece was Ophelia's speech to Laertes. In a raw and broken whisper, she starts reciting Shakespeare:

There's rosemary,
that's for remembrance.
Pray you, love, remember.
And there's pansies, that's for thoughts . . .

Her monologue is cut short by the cough. When it passes I ask, 'Did you get in?'

'I was accepted but not for the scholarship. It was after my mother died and an aunt, who was looking after me, said, "Oh you can't go on the stage, dear. It would break your mother's heart." I think she meant that it would break *her* heart. Actresses weren't exactly scarlet women then but you wouldn't have them around for tea.'

'So you joined your father's bank.'

'And hated it.'

Katrin cooks dinner for two. We need no longer tailor our menu to Mum's tastes because she eats next to nothing. Over roast vegetables I ask Katrin what she'd like to do this evening.

'Go out for a few drinks and then supper.'

I open a second bottle of wine. I type these words, drunk, until I start pressing the wrong keys and deleting paragraphs. Next door, Mum's cough breaks blood vessels in her eyes. I increase her morphine and she frets about her constipation.

'I've had no action in two days,' she complains.

'That's because you haven't eaten anything.'

'So what am I going to do?'

'I don't know. I'm sorry. I don't know.'

The predicted storm finally reaches the village. As the electricity fails, Mum has a terrible, uncontrollable coughing fit. We run to her by candlelight. I pour out more morphine and wine. We kneel beside her, each holding a hand. Katrin tells her to think of lavender fields, to feel the sun on her head, on the tips of her ears. I realize I'm ready for her to die, to stop breathing even as I feel her pulse beating in her wrist. I tell her not to talk, that we are with her. I don't understand how she can still be coughing. She is awash with morphine.

She doesn't die. The fit passes. She needs to lie down. We try to position her on her side in bed, settling her hips in the middle of the mattress. She can't find a familiar, comfortable position because her 'tired, old body' has changed. But within seconds she's asleep. Outside the thunder clouds roll along the far line of hills.

Monday 8th

Rory: 'See you next week, all being well,' carer Pauline calls from the door. Florence Nightingale says, 'I don't know if I'll see you – sorry, *when* I'll see you – again.' An off-duty nurse phones to ask if she can drop by 'to say hello'. Meaning to say goodbye.

'Do you remember Joan?' Katrin asks Rosie, the

precocious three-year-old daughter of a friend. 'Will you give Joan a kiss?'

'No but I'm going to jump on her bed,' Rosie announces, promptly throwing the pillows on to the floor.

'You're a very beautiful girl,' Mum tells her.

'And adorable, too,' she adds before running up and down the hall, crying, 'It's too late. It's too late.'

Today Mum eats a scoop of ice cream and a corner of salmon fillet. She drinks half a mug of cranberry juice, a glass of water and a cup of coffee. She sits in her chair, neither reading nor sorting, unable to do her nails because her hands are shaking too much. She tries to write in her diary, leaving barely legible scratches across the page. She tries to fold a sheet of paper and slip it into an envelope but reduces it instead to a crumpled ball.

Joan: R read us good draft of his festival talk with props – came in wearing safari hat, knapsack over shoulder to speak 'on why travel writers never leave home'. In knapsack he has slippers, pouring out cuppa – funny opening to supposedly serious talk. K shortened and shaped my nails, thoughtfully bought me Floradix for strength. I discovered new position to sit in chair – much more relaxed and comfortable. M is back in Marrakech. She's home from honeymoon tomorrow.

Rory: 'Darling, what's happening?'

Mum's left arm is twitching violently. Steroids reduce cerebral inflammation so I run to my study to get a pill, spilling the contents of the bottle across my desk. By the time I'm back her whole body is jerking in a heart-beat rhythm.

'Oh darling . . .'

She can't swallow the pill. I manage to get water into her mouth. I hold her hand. After a terrible minute the shaking stops.

Tuesday 9th

Rory: At dawn the village seems to have vanished. The misty air is cool, damp and still. Mum glances out at the indistinct world, raising her hands as if to part the clouds. 'It's ominous,' she tells us. Katrin closes the window. Last night she dreamed of holding her, crying, saying goodbye.

Today Mum is even weaker, unable to hold herself erect. I strain my back while helping her to her feet. Denise, this morning's carer, washes her as she sits astride Lightning. When we're alone, she tells me that carers often go home at the end of their shift and weep. I tell her that I can't read the signs any more.

'Take each day as it comes, sweetheart. Each day as it comes.'

When Mum lays herself back on the bed, the light seems to have gone from her eyes.

I help the *Sunday Times* find photos of mermaids and await a call from *Publishing News*. During the telephone interview, I step out into the hall from time to time, watching Mum sleep, listening for her breath.

'So where to next?' asks the chirpy interviewer. 'Have you started work on the next book?'

I'm coy and tell him nothing. But afterwards I'm troubled by my reticence and ring him back.

'Rodney, I don't want to be disingenuous with you. I did

start a new travel book but then my mother was diagnosed with cancer. I've stopped working on it to look after her.'

He tells me that his wife's mother is also dying of cancer.

Next CancerCare Carole telephones us. I tell her about last night's convulsions as well as the loss of appetite and strength, the indigestion, the five or six minutes coughing every hour. She explains how the steroids are both weakening Mum and keeping her alive.

'You and Katrin have to consider this dilemma,' she says.

'We can still cope with her here,' I reassure her, thinking that she is reminding us of the hospice.

'That's not what I mean,' she replies.

At first I don't get it. Then I understand. For four months the steroids have kept the symptoms under control. But now the cancer is so advanced that we need to decide whether to increase them, or withdraw them.

Later, minister John drops by the house. Mum thanks him for the plant.

'I was brought up to bring ladies flowers,' he tells her.

'I need to ask you something,' she says to him, taking his hand. 'And maybe I shouldn't be asking a minister this.'

'We're quite used to hearing a lot of peculiar things.'

'I can't believe in the Bible as fact and a grey-haired man sitting on a throne dispensing judgement and thunderbolts.'

Wednesday 10th

Joan: Awoke 7.15. V. difficult to sit up – definitely going downhill as R had to help me. Yesterday, John said, 'Belief in Bible and God doesn't matter as long as one has faith in love and the power of love.' Glad to have cleared this up.

Rory: In the cool light of morning I sit holding my crying mother's hand.

'The situation is difficult to accept when one's been used to getting on with life,' she says, tears rolling down her face, plopping on the blackcurrant stain on her nightie.

I decide to miss my Wednesday morning swim. I don't feel able to leave her today. Downstairs, Katrin feeds the dog before going to the pool. As she puts the bowl on the floor, Tess lunges at her, ripping her shirt. Katrin screams and falls back, slamming the door on her.

Breakfast is a frothy energy drink; nuts, honey, yoghurt and Providextra. Over the course of the morning Mum drinks half the mug. At lunchtime I warm up yesterday's salmon. It tastes like airline food.

'Where's the dinner tray?' I ask Katrin.

'I put it away,' she says. 'We only carry up single plates now.'

I take the fish to Mum. Spread across the table in front of her are my father's love letters.

'I'm not reading them. Only putting them in date order.'

She promises to eat the fillet but only manages two small flakes and a single green bean.

The cough returns at the same time as CancerCare Carole. Another dose of Oramorph enables them to talk. Carole likens energy to a commodity. I ask her about the wisdom of keeping next week's appointment with Dr Marsden. The trip to Dorchester would exhaust her and there is nothing more to do, or say.

'Do you want to go?' she asks Mum.

'He will want to see me,' she answers, clinging on to me

and the idea. 'He'll want to take a new X-ray to evaluate my progress.'

Carole proposes a compromise. 'I'll ring and ask him to look at the last X-ray, to see if that gives him enough information for the moment. Then, if it does, we could make a later appointment.'

Mum nods in acceptance, then asks, 'Do you want to see Marlie's wedding photos?'

At the front door Carole tells me she wants a doctor to check the leg sores, which are now in danger of becoming infected. In her appointment diary I see that another patient's name has been crossed out on page after page. Carole also prescribes three new drugs; one to counter the indigestion, another to suppress the cough, plus a glycerine spray more helpful in stopping the mouth from drying.

'And the steroids?' I ask. 'Can I keep increasing the dosage?'

'Until they lose their effectiveness.'

'Then what do we do?'

'We use sedatives,' says Carole.

Thursday 11th

Joan: Awake at 5.55 a.m. but without the ability to stand and move to armchair. Fortunately, R has early departure so I'm in armchair now. Yesterday I had to remind Florence to look at my leg, which she bandaged as sore leaking. I asked Carole to stop Florence's visits. I said a change would be a compassionate and practical solution, neither of which qualities that hopeless woman has shown me. Carole will investigate. She will also check with Dr

Marsden whether it is essential that he sees me next Friday as planned.

K to collect M from station at lunchtime today. I've asked her to warn M of my decline in health.

Rory: I don't know how many people are sleeping in the house. Has Marlie arrived yet? Are Andrew, Margaret and Neal still upstairs in the attic? I don't feel that it's just the three of us here. We have had many visitors but this is different. I sense another presence, and imagine again that my father's spirit has entered the house.

I have to be away from home today. I'm due to give a talk at the Swindon Book Festival. I'm up early to help Mum to her chair. On our journey she needs to pause twice, catching her breath at the edge of the bed, before reaching her chair. I'm anxious that she might die in the six hours I'm away.

As I drive off, a needling wind blows up, brushing blossoms down the lane and spitting raindrops on my windshield. The road to Swindon is long. I eat an egg mayonnaise sandwich in the car. I have an audience of thirty-five; small but not disappointing because of their thoughtful questions. On the drive back to Dorset I find myself singing along to *Evita* on the radio – '. . . that I'm immune to gloom, that I'm hard through and through . . .'

At home, Marlie has arrived, bringing dusty red roses from Marrakech.

'I never thought I'd be given flowers from Morocco,' says Mum, excited by her return. Her whole lower leg – from knee to ankle – is now dressed in a bandage.

Over dinner downstairs we talk about the steroids' diminishing effectiveness at containing the brain inflammation. Changing her dosage could make the difference between a sudden, painful end and a slow, numb death.

'But the next time she has a fit, I'll have to give her even more steroids,' I say to Marlie.

'Maybe just going to sleep – on the long course of sedatives – is the most humane way.'

Friday 12th

Rory: At seven I push open her door. Mum is lying on her back. 'I can't sit up,' she says, close to tears. She's unable to reach the bedside table, turn on the lamp, look at the time. Her last independence is lost. 'I can't get myself to the edge of the bed.'

I try to make light of this morning's development. 'I can lift you. That's no problem.'

'It's not a long-term solution.'

Marlie and Katrin come into the room.

'We have to have a family conference,' announces Mum, staring up at the ceiling. 'I can't get up without help.'

'Isn't that why you had us?' teases Marlie. 'To look after you in your old age.'

Mum seems to have developed a new tremor in her hands, though the shaking might only be in my imagination. She drinks her seed laxative for breakfast, then coughs up much of it. The colour drains out of her face. Her mauve jumper looks like a mucky bib.

Thankfully, Marlie does all the caring today, enabling me at least to finish my tax return. Our GP calls in from the surgery. She is kind, helpful and confident. Her presence reassures Mum. Then at the front door she says to me, 'There comes a time when there's not much more that we can do.' Mike arrives from London with the wedding and honeymoon videos. We connect their camera to the television and the light and noise of Morocco blaze into the bedroom. Katrin and I seize the chance to go to a dinner party, reaching our friends' house at eight and hurrying back by ten in order to see Mum before bedtime.

Joan: First anniversary of Marlie meeting Mike. They play me audio-video of wedding – heard their pledge to one another – wonderful to hear. Some confusion over picture of a woman while voice of a man recorded at same time. In need of editing.

Sunday 14th

Rory: On Saturday Marlie tended to Mum's needs again. Katrin dreamed of Mum as a wrinkled baby, then went to work. I drove to Sherborne to buy her birthday present. After lunch, Mike and I did the dishes, talking about science and sacrifice, my next book and his upcoming lecture. Marlie sat at Mum's feet, her head on her lap. At five the newlyweds headed back to London. In the evening Katrin joined friends at the Sherborne Real Ale Festival. I left home only for fifteen minutes to collect my laughing, drunken wife.

Today we're awoken early by the sound of crop sprayers, not cuckoos. The hazy morning promises another hot afternoon. Again Mum's room is in darkness. Only the end of her bed is visible through the half-open door and her feet are still. I peer around the door. Mum looks up at me, unable to lift her disintegrating body from the bed. Her eyes are huge, distressed, alive.

'Please help me up.'

I put one arm under her shoulders, the other under her knees and swivel her to the side of the bed. The effort winds her.

'Just let me catch my breath.'

She's gasping. She can't get enough oxygen. It's sixty seconds before she can say, 'I don't think I can reach the chair.'

'Carole said that you could spend more time in bed,' I remind her.

She nods, surrendering another ounce of resolve, and allows me to lay her back down.

When I return to bed, Katrin says, 'I thought you'd left me alone again.'

Joan: Slept till 8.30 a.m. Sat up but didn't have strength to stand so laid down until carer arrived at 10.30 and dozed, then much more rested. R saying, 'Take each day as it comes,' which I'm sure is right.

Rory: We're tired, by the emotion, by the sameness of caring, by the boredom of routine. Death need not be dramatic; there may be no insight or profundity, only repetition. Our Sunday vanishes in petty tasks and small gestures; dispensing yoghurt-nut drink, adjusting pillows. Katrin plants basil seeds. I put the Zimmer frame away in the garage. Mum eats a bowl of ice cream.

We want to show her the garden in the evening light. She hasn't looked out on to it for a week, so we wheel her to our bedroom window. She stands up, her shaking hands grasping my arm, her breath coming in gasps. Once she feared falling down the stairs. Now she dreads falling when standing.

'So much has changed.'

'The wisteria is out.'

'Where?'

'Just beyond the veronica, and the purple geranium from your garden.'

She and Katrin talk about the prunus and the japonica. When the evening's carer arrives, we help her to undress Mum. Katrin needs to shove her left foot back so she can sit on Lightning. All the while, Mum's eyes never leave the garden. I wheel her back to the bedside and she asks, 'What are we doing now?'

'Now we're going to bed.'

Katrin and I help her to stand and then to sit on the bed. I give her two Temazepam and rest her head on the pillow. I move her hips and shoulders into a comfortable position as she can no longer do so herself. Two of us are needed to move her. I kiss her forehead and tell her that she is precious.

'Lucky me. That's four times today.'

In the hall I blow my nose.

'Are you all right?' she asks from the dark bedroom.

'I just blew my nose.'

'I thought I heard you call out.'

'I'm fine. Good night.'

Monday 15th

Rory: 'I want to sit up,' says Mum. 'How do we do it?'

This morning Katrin pulls a muscle while lifting her to the chair. Once again I'm gripped by anger, which simmers in me for much of the morning. In my study I cast out abandoned projects, collate untyped notes, smile when Mum calls me back to her room to pick up a dropped pen or diary (she's transcribing extracts from a book on Leonardo da Vinci). I don't want her to feel any sense of imposition or guilt. But at midmorning she asks about Katrin's back and Katrin won't lie, changing the conversation instead of answering her. Then as we sip miso soup, Mum needs to go to the loo. Her stomach is upset and she needs to be returned to the bathroom four times over the next two hours. She writes down the times of her bowel movements. Katrin tells her to stop torturing herself.

In the garden Katrin finds herself singing Terry Jacks' 'Seasons in the Sun' about saying goodbye when the birds are singing in the sky.

'This is no time to die,' she tells me, blinking in the sun. 'When it's so sunny and beautiful.'

'It's the best time to die. Not in the depths of winter. Now, with the world so alive.'

Around three o'clock Mum asks to be put to bed. I lay her down and pull the blind. She looks up at me.

'I'd like to go to the hospice please,' she says, 'and I don't want you to feel that you've failed.'

'We can look after you, Mum.'

'I've been trembling again down my left-hand side. I'm going downhill faster than I expected. In a week or two I'll die. So it doesn't really matter if I go now or in a few days.'

I'm holding her hand. Her skin is soft. I remind her that we could have lost her years ago, as she lost her mother. I watch my verb tenses when we speak now; 'we have this time together' not 'we've had this time together'. I ask her if she wants to die alone. She doesn't.

'But it can't be easy on Katrin. I'm her mother-*in-law*. And I don't want to continue upsetting your routine.'

She insists that we discuss her moving out. When I do,

Katrin responds, 'If she dies somewhere else, I'll feel so cheated.' We began an emotional journey in undertaking to care for Mum until the end. If she goes to the hospice, we reason, it would be out of consideration for us.

Katrin makes milky coffee and two big mugs of tea. I carry the tray and a new packet of biscuits. We sit on the bedroom floor, telling her that we want her to stay in our house.

'Our lives will be more disrupted if you move out,' says Katrin, following the strategy we've agreed to adopt.

'With you at home we can work a little, answer the phone, I can write my journal,' I say. 'If you move into a hospice, we'll spend hours driving back and forth.'

'I hadn't thought of that,' she says, closing her eyes with exhaustion and relief.

'We want you to stay where you feel safe and loved.'

'You can die here, Mum,' I say.

In the evening she brushes her teeth for fifteen minutes, until droplets of blood spot the porcelain sink.

'What are you doing?' I ask.

'I'm trying to get the food out from between my teeth.'

'You've only eaten two spoonfuls of porridge today, Mum. Nothing is caught between your teeth.'

Joan: 'He who wishes to see how the soul inhabits the body should look to see how that body uses its daily surroundings. If the body is dirty and neglected, the body will be kept by its soul in the same condition, dirty and neglected.'

I imagine Leonardo being fanatical about cleanliness. In the middle of a recipe for mixing pigments he wrote, 'take some fresh water and moisten your hands with it then some lavender flowers and rub them between your palms.'

Tuesday 16th – Katrin's birthday

Rory: If time stands still, how can Katrin have reached her birthday? While she walks Tess, I arrange on the kitchen table cards, candles and presents: a Design Museum catalogue from her mother, a pocket camera from me. Upstairs she opens Mum's gift: a Museum of Modern Art anthology of nature poetry. In it she has written, 'May you continue to bring joy to those whose lives you touch and find even greater joy in your own life.'

I cook a prawn biriani birthday supper. We plan to watch *Anna Karenina* on television. I make a duck-egg omelette for Mum but she needs the loo as soon as I bring it. She tenses herself, despairs; we're too late. Katrin changes her pad. I wheel her back to her bedroom then reheat the omelette. 'I haven't had a duck egg since the war,' she says, trying to enthuse. Her indigestion returns after two forkfuls. I administer Gaviscon liquid to neutralize the acid in her shrunken stomach and take away her plate. 'But it's so delicious,' she pleads. We've missed the beginning of the film. Then the family calls to wish Katrin happy birthday.

'I've asked her to buy me an electric toothbrush,' Mum tells me. I don't know what I am going to do with the teeth in the refrigerator.

Anna Karenina ends while we're laying Mum down in bed. She tenses as I try to move her into a comfortable position. I tell her to relax. Again she tenses. Katrin's temper begins to fray.

'Be a sack of potatoes, Mum.'

'I don't know why I'm doing it.'

Impatiently I push her into position, against her tension. I kiss her perfunctorily and turn out the light.

In bed Katrin asks me, 'Is there anything that you want to say to your Mum?'

Wednesday 17th

Rory: Katrin and I stand at our bedroom window, looking out on the garden. A grey cap of dawn cloud covers the village until the sun glints orange through a tear in the sky and adorns St Andrew's in radiance.

'I'm going to tell her to stop fighting,' I say.

This morning Mum couldn't find the button on her electric blanket. She couldn't read the clock. Her eyes were the colour of warm milk. She told me, more from reflex than out of conviction, 'If I don't get up, I'll make no progress.'

I tell her to stay longer in bed. She takes it as her cue. I lean her back on to the pillows. I set the armchair beside her and sit in it. After she has caught her breath I repeat my belief that she will always be with me.

'I was just about to say the same thing. I believe it.'

'Andrew believes that he can find you through prayer. Marlie will find a way, too.'

'I think she's looking now.'

'So you needn't worry about us, Mum,' I tell her. 'You can let go.'

'I'm not worried, darling. May I have another drink?'

I hold the cup to her lips. We spill a little tea.

'John has been talking about the Bible. I can't go along with everything he says.'

'His point is that dying isn't an end.'

'It's just another stage of life,' says Mum. 'A new chapter.' House martins fly up past the window, to their nests under the eaves. She takes my hand. 'You are my young angels, and I'm surrounded by the spirits of others.'

I ask who she feels around us. My father? Her parents? 'I suppose we need to learn to differentiate between angels,' I say.

She sleeps. Her breathing is dry then wet. I listen to the clock ticking on the window sill. When she starts to cough, I wonder if this is the moment to withhold the steroids, for *me* to stop fighting and to let her go.

Friday 19th

Rory: Yesterday Mum seemed stronger. Today she stays in bed until noon. Yesterday she asked me about the publicity plans for *Next Exit Magic Kingdom*. Today she seems halfway there herself. Her eyes are heavy, her speech is slurred, her mouth so dry that I need to spray it with artificial saliva every few minutes. Carole asks her, 'Are you frightened of dying?'

'I'm frightened about my death hurting those who care about me. I think it's better that I die alone to spare them the pain.'

'But surely Rory, Marlie and Katrin will want to be with you at the end.'

'I hadn't thought of that.'

'There's been a lot for you to accept,' Carole tells Mum.

'Yes there has, Carole. Thank you.'

Yesterday morning Mum watched the European Grand Prix trials from the Nürburgring. This afternoon she learns to fly. To help us lift her in and out of bed – and to protect our backs – a great, white, wheeled Oxford crane is delivered by social services. We slip her into its sling to swing her between bed and chair. She beams like a baby, making us laugh, calling out, 'I'm airborne! I'm flying!' I make whirring aircraft noises to the delight of our Magnificent Woman in Her Flying Machine.

Joan: Helen brought lift – hilarious Ealing comedy as both R and I have rides in hoist – pleasantly best just to relax back with hands resting on thighs and let hoist do the work. Will ease young angels' backs hopefully. Jane, who is very compassionate, urges me not to rush. Carole asking if I fear death – 'I was just wondering?' – too hard on myself.

Hakkinen is narrowing the points gap on Schumacher. At last.

Saturday 20th

Katrin: Marlie is down for the weekend so Rory and I escaped, heading down to the coast (to anywhere with a vantage point) with my birthday present from him. Maybe because of the new camera, our walk has already become a series of static images, frozen in memory. I was busy looking through the viewfinder, experimenting with the different formats, framing images, focusing on details: hanging fields above a cliff edge, a scoop of land beyond which lay the sea, a field punctuated by a single, bent tree, shaped by the prevailing wind, myself beneath a signpost – caught in panoramic format – arms spread wide, to east and west. Clear, brisk, bright weather.

Knowing that Joan is about to die gives another dimension to this collage of impressions, magnifying them and imbuing them with a lasting clarity. I am keenly aware of a new and vivid quality to everything around me and of seeing the world with a startling blend of detachment and immediacy. As we walk up Goldencap through fields of orchids in the May sunshine, I sense that every detail of this precious present is being sharply etched in my mind.

Having anticipated – and imagined – Joan's death for so long, I already see our vital present as history. As the end approaches, I am looking back to the way we were – the way we are – when she was still alive, surveyed as if from the future, even now, this very instant, as I am still within it. Moment by moment we are all sliding towards the same vanishing point, knowing that at the moment of transition – when we cross the threshold and begin to move *away from* rather than *towards* – the sum of our experience will be reduced to memory alone.

Sunday 21st

Rory: On Friday I dreamed of falling off a cliff. Yesterday I walked along the edge of the Dorset coastal path.

When we returned home from Goldencap, Mum was still in bed. She acknowledged she's most relaxed lying down.

Katrin conjured up grilled peppers and feta for lunch. Mum unexpectedly gobbled it up as Marlie and I found ourselves back in Canada. Unconsciously, my sister said 'furnace room' instead of 'utility room'. I used 'elevator' rather than 'lift'. At the shop I asked for two per cent milk rather than semi-skimmed.

Mum was also reaching for the reassurance of childhood memories.

'When I'm uncomfortable, I don't think of Canada any more. I've started picturing my father's bluebell wood. It came to me quite suddenly. He loved that wood. It was right next door to our house in Esher.'

This morning a soft rain falls in billowing sheets. The

hills vanish behind the clouds as the peonies raise their heads towards the sky. I'm up at five, six and seven. First, Mum coughs in her sleep. I try to give her morphine but she winces when I move her, so I slip a Lorazepam under her tongue. The second time she calls – she can no longer reach the bedside bell – to ask me to rub foot lotion into her heels. 'They feel so burnt and raw.' The skin is cool to the touch. The third time she is having difficulty breathing. Her moss green eyes have dulled to khaki.

I mix Maxijul into her morning cranberry drink, then Marlie and I sit by her bedside, talking about journeys.

'Italy will be beautiful in July,' says Mum.

'Mike and I hope to go to France in August.'

'Mum, when you're off on your travels, don't think that you always have to watch over us. There will be lots of other things you'll need to do.'

'Just keep speaking to me,' she replies. 'I'll be listening.'

As we talk, she begins to slur her words. She misses her mouth when lifting a glass of soda water to her lips. I notice that her fingers have begun to swell around her wedding ring. One blessing of a slow death is that one has time to begin to accept inevitable changes.

In the afternoon Marlie has to catch her train back to London. Mum holds her hand and says, 'We've had quite an adventure, haven't we, darling?' They kiss goodbye. 'See you next weekend.'

'I hope so but if you want to go before then, do go,' says Marlie.

'I'm not ready to go to the bluebell wood yet,' she answers, casually. 'Mind you, I haven't done this before.'

While Katrin runs Marlie to the station, I sit with Mum, now tossing her head from time to time and releasing an inward moan.

'What's happening?' I ask her. I want to know.

'I don't know yet,' she manages to reply, squeezing my hand.

And I laugh. I feel joy for her and the journey she's about to begin.

Monday 22nd

Rory: I'm waiting for the kettle to boil when Tess stares at me and walks to the bottom of the steps. I bolt upstairs, ease open Mum's door and call her name. Her eyes are closed. I don't hear her breathing. I repeat her name.

'Mum?'

'Yes, darling?' She opens her eyes. Her diary is beside her.

'I . . . I was wondering if you'd like coffee or hot chocolate this afternoon.'

Joan: Sweet call from A in Canada – 'I couldn't miss chance to say we love you' – I asked him to tell Margaret how much we all appreciated her make-up of our faces for the wedding. M back to work. R busy writing. John quite helpful with blessing.

– Love is a habit of the heart.
– As if all the time encircled by angels.
– Nothing unlovely in the world.

Rory: I try to finish an article. The last sentence is incomplete. I can't get the tense right; present or past. I go out to record an interview with RTE, speaking from a local radio studio to Dublin about Disney World. I return to a house filled with the heady scent of summer. Katrin is making elderflower cordial. Her period is ten days late.

Tuesday 23rd – Thursday 25th

Rory: Katrin wakes with a heavy weight across her chest. Tess vomits on the kitchen floor. Mum hasn't the strength to open her diary. This morning's carer washes her in bed. I put the old bicycle horn by her hand again. She toots it every ten minutes, then every five, because of a pain in her shoulder, to ask me to adjust the pillows, for a drink. She opens her mouth but doesn't close it, even as I touch the straw to her lips.

'Close your mouth, Mum. Now suck.'

She moves herself up and down in the bed, adjusting its height with a new piece of equipment, unable to get comfortable.

'That's not bad,' she says, then changes her position again.

She asks me to straighten her legs. When I try to move them, she tenses, now fearful of falling even while lying flat on her back.

'Please try to relax.' She makes herself go limp but, as I start to lift her, she tenses again.

I feed her yoghurt so she can swallow her three steroid pills. Katrin massages Tiger Balm into her sore muscles.

'Are you all right?' I ask in a ridiculous, automatic mantra.

She grunts under her breath, 'I don't know.'

I sit by the bed all morning. Around noon I move her to the chair but immediately her neck starts to ache. She cannot settle no matter how I arrange the cushions behind her head. I exchange emails with Andrew and Marlie about the funeral. I update this diary entry, lie on the floor of my study and wait. Downstairs, Katrin telephones her friend Christine. When I cannot hear her voice, I know that she's crying.

'Oh God,' Mum moans and asks to go back in bed.

Katrin and I lift her with the hoist, my aircraft sounds evoking no smiles. I sit beside her once more.

'I'm here with you, Mum.'

'I know.'

Florence rings the bell. She's alarmed by the sudden change. She and Katrin insert a catheter. Mum breathes through her open mouth, hardly conscious.

CancerCare Carole tells us three to four days. I see no sense in increasing the steroids. We will put Mum on a drip tomorrow – if she lives until then. Carole asks if we can cope.

'Katrin,' I call out, cackling madly, 'can we cope?'

Mum starts to thrash in bed. Her breathing becomes laboured as if she's physically fighting. Carole thinks it's the brain tumour. She leaves and returns ten minutes later with half a vial of sedative from the surgery. Both Andrew and Marlie have agreed it's the kindest option. We try to discuss it with Mum but her eyes remain closed.

'I think it's for the best, Mum.'

'Fine, darling.'

Then as she drifts from consciousness again, she calls in a tender, loving voice, 'Andrew. Andrew.' My brother's name. My father's name.

Katrin cooks pasta and we eat it in the bedroom, sitting beside her, stroking her hands when she whimpers, without any sense of the morbid. I look at her – mouth open, cavities showing, catheter attached, dying – and am filled with a rush of love.

We decide to share the night in three-hour shifts. I go to bed first only to wake in an hour – just after midnight – when Mum has another panic attack. Wordlessly, she struggles to get out of bed. Katrin and I lift her to her feet but she doesn't want to sit on Lightning. She wants to stand with her arms around me. I hold her there, perhaps for the last time. Then I lower her into the chair. She scrabbles, eyes closed, fighting to move, fighting against being still. Minutes later we winch her back into bed. She gulps the air, five maybe six times, then collapses into exhaustion. Her pulse fades for seven . . . eight seconds. Then she suddenly gasps and grips my hand. Through the soft warm fold of her hand I feel her heart racing. Her stomach rumbles loudly beneath the duvet.

Katrin sleeps for an hour. I do the same. At four o'clock Mum is thrashing again. Neither the Lorazepam nor the Oramorph – which even a day ago seemed strong – have any effect. I call the duty doctor. He arrives after a long twenty-five minutes. I should have called him earlier.

He injects the remaining half ampoule of sedative. He writes on my list of drugs, 'Needs pump NOW.'

Katrin sleeps two more hours. Mum's nose and fingertips are blue. With her lids shut she asks me, 'Are you there now, darling?' then 'Shall we do what we were doing before?' then 'Just push.'

'What would you like me to push, Mum?'

'Anything. Just anything.'

I can't figure it out. Perhaps she's telling me to raise the bed's new electric backrest.

'Push the button?' I ask, triumphant, powering her up and down. But she has drifted away again. Did she mean push me back up the slope, the slippery slope and into a healthy life?

CancerCare Carole returns at nine o'clock Wednesday morning. No drug can ease the cerebral irritation.

'Poor love,' she says, connecting the syringe-driver pump to deliver her medication: Diamorphine 30 milligrams, Hypnorel 20 milligrams, Hyoscine 800 milligrams. She crushes two Dexamethasone tablets, mixes them with water and holding up her head manages to wash them down Mum's throat.

I try to encourage Mum to sip on a glass of water. She's had no liquid in twenty hours. Her eyes roll open for only a few sightless seconds.

'I feel awful,' she says, then, 'Thank you, Katrin dear,' then 'Mummy! Mummy!' She calls my name when I'm in the bathroom. I run in to find her eyes firmly shut. I can't go downstairs. I can hardly leave the room.

Minister John is in the chapel allotment when I call him. At our door he hands me a muddy, freshly picked lettuce, then stands at the end of the bed to pray for God's help to let her go easily into His care.

I ring Andrew and Marlie, who leaves the office at lunchtime. At five, when she reaches us, Mum is too doped to squeeze her right hand; that's better than pain. Marlie sits holding her hand, telling her about her day, crying.

Now there are three of us to divide the night. We agree on a shared watch of ninety-minute shifts: 10.30 to midnight to 1.30 to 3.00 to 4.30. Marlie is first followed by me at midnight. I hold Mum's hand but there is no sign that she knows I'm with her. To keep awake I read a ludicrous article in *Marie Claire* on sleep deprivation and cancer.

'On the day after a sleepless night, there may be fewer cancer-fighting cells available to fight off invaders. In one study, people who stayed up until 3 a.m. had 30 per cent fewer natural cancer-killing cells the next day.'

I wake Katrin and go back to bed.

At 4.30 on Thursday morning I take over from Marlie. She says 'No change' but Mum's pulse, when I can find it, is frail. Through the course of the night her breathing has become thick and laboured. Last night's sharp intake of breath is replaced by a weary bluntness. Yesterday brought the realization that she might not speak again. This morning I understand that the bright spark of her spirit will never shine on me again, at least not this side of death.

Beside her, I flick through yesterday's post. An investment flyer encourages me 'to look into the huge financial potential of medicine'. As I'm reading it, her breath starts to whistle. The change startles me and I start to talk to her, about her stay with us, about the journey she's about to begin. I tell her that we are surrounded by love because she followed her heart all her life.

And she squeezes my hand.

So I keep talking. I say that her mother and my father are waiting for her in the bluebell wood (now enhanced with Canadian silver birches), that I look forward to seeing her again, that I'll almost live for the reunion, someday, somehow.

And she opens her eyes.

I talk on, talking for us both. I tell her that I feel deep sadness for the loss of her, but real joy for her new beginning. She seems to be clinging to such a thin thread. I massage her shoulders. When she starts to wheeze, I run and wake Katrin who wakes Marlie. Mum opens her eyes, sees her daughter and says, 'Darling Marlie, how lovely that you've come.'

We surround the bed, sitting beside her, giving her drops

of water by eye-dropper. She keeps placing her hand on her poor swollen belly. We stroke it, the cancer.

Marlie tells her that she is beautiful. Katrin says, 'Go softly.' I repeat, 'We're here.' Meaning that she's still here.

'I know. Thank you, darlings.'

It feels like the end. Minutes pass. Mum closes her eyes. Our limbs become cramped. I stand and stretch. We change positions. Marlie puts moisturizer on Mum's face. Katrin calls the shop to say she's not coming in to work. Her period starts, twelve days late. I wind my desk clock, the one Mum gave me when I first left Canada, and I've kept running these last five months. Again and again we think she is about to die. We want it to end. We want to relieve her, to relieve us, but she clings on, surfacing briefly – and weirdly – then sinking back into unconsciousness.

'I feel old,' she says.

At ten when Carole arrives, Mum looks better.

'Her pulse is strong,' she says.

She increases the painkiller and Mum falls back into a deep, drugged sleep. Her objective is to slow the brain as the body dies. She writes in her report, 'Calm and peaceful but may have some pain. Diamorphine increased to 40 milligrams. Hyoscine given by I.M. May need Midazolam (Hypnovel) increase tomorrow, in which case two pumps will be needed.' The hoist sits on the landing like some long-necked, prehistoric monster with a white sling across its shoulder. In the doorway Carole tells me about the procedure for reporting a death.

The afternoon slips away. Katrin moistens Mum's mouth with lemon and glycerine swabs. I drip more water on to her tongue. Marlie massages her feet. Her face becomes very red, almost florid, her skin clammy; her heart pumps on in her motionless body. I try to nap but a sudden rainstorm wakes me, washing the heat out of a sunny day.

Later, Katrin and I walk around the village. When we return, I pick up the kitchen kettle. Its handle smells of Mum's hand lotion. How could she have come downstairs? Then I realize that Marlie had used her lotion.

Friday 26th

Rory: Wet and miserable day. The wind rages at the windows. No time to 'go gentle into that good night'. Mike – who arrived at midnight – shakes me out of a dream about dividing eternity into ninety-minute segments. Now we are four, plus one.

Two new district nurses stomp through the front door, leaving wet footprints along the hallway. They come to clean and care, rolling Mum on to her side while I squeeze her hand and feel her quake. Her pulse is alternatively robust then barely detectable. Her mouth is clotted with thrush. Since Wednesday she's had no more than a few teaspoons of liquid. Marlie washes her face and hands with a face cloth. In the afternoon she focuses on Katrin and says, 'Mummy.' Her breath smells putrid.

I stay inside all day, taking calls and editing the *Sunday Times* extract. Next week I begin my publicity tour, which includes a TV appearance. Today I can't even look at myself in the mirror.

When we are downstairs the mains are cut and I run upstairs, sure that she is gone. But Mum sleeps on. When the electricity is restored my father's duck lamp fuses beside her bed. Years ago he had made it for her from a wooden decoy. I check the bulb, the fuse and the wires. There is no reason for it not to work.

Saturday 27th

Rory: Today dawns with a high, cloudless blue sky. The air is cool and fresh, washed clean by yesterday's rain. Katrin, who shared the night watch with Mike and Marlie, takes a shower. She's working today. The three of them left me undisturbed in a deep, dreamless sleep. I take Tess for a walk. There are birds singing in the hedgerows. I hear over and over in my head, 'A beautiful day to die. A beautiful day to die.'

Back home I make our bed, shower and change my clothes. I pack the remaining drugs into two plastic bags to return to the dispensary. Lightning, the walking frame, the hoist and bed riser must all go back to social services, along with the hospital table, which was dropped off on Monday in the rain, never to be used. The bathroom looks bare since Katrin removed the extra towels.

I sit by the bed with my laptop, looking at my mother. She lies on her side, unmoved and unmoving for twenty-four hours. Her gentle, closed eyes are clean now, Marlie having sponged away the sleep. Her skin is English rose, neither florid nor pale. Her cheeks are hollow. Her thin, grey hair curves down around her neck to the point where I watch her pulse. Her jaw twists open with every wet, muffled breath. We're told she can't feel any pain. She looks peaceful in her last, deep sleep.

Marlie buys cheese and ham from Oak House Stores. I make a salad. Katrin calls twice from the shop to ask, 'Any change?' I ring Andrew in Canada. Marlie, Mike and I sit on the landing, eating, talking, reading the paper. I take her address book – the one I bought her last year in Siena – and draw up a list of friends to call. The house smells of lavender, face cream and antiseptic.

Then I glance at Mum. The colour has drained from her

face. Her skin is the colour of porcelain. I call Katrin at work. Her boss answers the phone.

'Has she . . . ?' asks Vicky.

Katrin is with a customer.

'Mum's still here,' I say. 'But there are a few signs. Can you ask her to call me?'

Vicky doesn't give Katrin the message.

Suddenly the foam in Mum's mouth is thicker. As Marlie and I try to swab it out her breathing becomes shallower, more tenuous. The palms of her hands turn blue. I call the shop again. This time Katrin picks up the telephone.

'I'm coming.'

'Katrin, drive carefully.'

I run back to the bedroom. Mum has no strength left to cough so the foam swells into her mouth and over her lips. Marlie and I now use tissues to clear it away. She is crying, mopping, and I'm holding her hand, or Mike's or Mum's, I'm not sure. Mum's breathing seems to rise in her mouth, no deeper. It slows, stops for five seconds, is followed by another wet, foamy inhalation. Her eyelids open a fraction but not into consciousness. I see only the whites of her eyes. Mike searches for her pulse. The breath stops again.

All of a sudden Marlie is talking. She is telling Mum that we love her, that we'll remember all that she's taught us. I'm talking, too, telling her to go to the bluebell wood. I'm sure she can't hear us. It's maybe fifteen seconds since her last breath. There is no colour in her face. I want to say, 'Wait Mum, Katrin's coming.'

'She's still alive,' says Mike. 'She still has a pulse.'

A sudden, impertinent last breath and it's over. I may be wiping away foam. I may be holding her hand. Her eyelids may quiver. But I don't think so.

'Is there still a pulse?' I ask Mike.

If he answers, I don't hear him. There isn't another

breath. There is no single instant of death, or not one we can recognize. Mum dies over five or ten seconds, five months, eighty years. There is no opening of eyes, no final advice (her last word was 'Tha . . .' to Katrin in the night). I want to sense her spirit lift up out of her. I want to feel her go free. But I sense no change. The room feels the same. She is still a presence in the house, in our lives.

'Open the window,' says Marlie, to let her soul fly free.

We can't avert our eyes from her brave and dignified face. The foam stopped expanding with her breathing. I hold Marlie. We keep watching her. Mike hugs us. In the crook of the embrace I see my watch. Ten to three. Marlie is weeping.

I close Mum's eyelids.

'Carole told me to lay her out straight and put her head to one side to keep the mouth closed.'

I try to shut her mouth but it keeps falling open. We lift off the duvet and roll her on to her back. I arrange her warm limbs, her swollen knees, her puffy feet. Marlie straightens her arms. We cover her body again. We stroke her hair, her cheek. I hear our car drive up – fast. I go downstairs. Through the glass I see Katrin fumbling for her key. I open the door and shake my head. She holds me tight in the hallway. We go upstairs. She is saying, 'Joan. Joan.'

Summers and Winters

Rory: Seven years on I clearly remember that first afternoon, and the feeling that you were still in your room, somewhere near the golden armchair.

'We can't come to you now,' an overworked nurse told me on the phone, her priorities shifting, her role to care for the living, not the departed. 'There aren't enough bodies around today.'

We knelt beside your body to say a prayer with John. A shadow fleeted across the bed and your hand didn't move. We cleaned away your drinking glass and damp tissues, changed the duvet for your pink blanket. Marlie and Mike removed your wedding ring from your blue fingers. We stroked your hair and kissed your still-warm forehead. I brought Tess upstairs but she was too excited to notice you, wagging her tail at the joy of being among the living.

Stan the jolly undertaker arrived at six, full of apologies for his delay. He'd been out walking in the hills and from them he gushed forth gales of laughter along with another story from beyond the grave.

'Did I tell you about the jealous sister who put her brother's share certificates in his coffin so his wife wouldn't inherit them?'

Only when his assistant brought up the stretcher and body bag did he become business-like again.

'This can't be done prettily, so would you mind leaving us alone?'

They zipped you into a black body bag and carried you

downstairs. At the front door I wondered aloud if I should ask for a receipt.

'I've never been asked for one of those before,' chuckled Stan.

Afterwards, we stripped the bed, loading the sheet and pillow cases into the washing machine. Marlie hoovered while Mike did the dishes. Outside Katrin clung to your duvet by the washing line. When I went to her she said, 'It smells of her. It all smells of her.' After supper Marlie and Mike drove back to London. Katrin and I went to bed. Sometime in the night I awoke from a dream of rolling you in – or unrolling you from – the roller blind.

The following morning in your room – the 'green room' again – we didn't remove your things as we'd planned. Instead, we changed the water in your flowers and lit a scented candle. The first condolence email arrived and I automatically printed it out to show it to you. In your bedside table, among the Fruit Pastilles and hairpins, I found an old notebook, which I'd never seen before. In it you had written three or four pages of quotations, probably when in your early thirties and on your way from the UK to Canada. Between your thoughts on identity ('freedom is not only self-expression, it is also self-control') and relationships ('the secret of love is communication'), you had written, 'I set out with the nebulous queasy feeling in my tummy which seems to accompany all adventures – whether physical or emotional – away from warm, comforting, known things.'

Forty-eight hours on, Stan rang to confirm the time of your cremation.

'I'll try not to be late,' he said, hoping to reassure me. 'But I have to MOT the hearse beforehand.'

Katrin: It was strange being able to go out when I wanted, without the need to plan or consult with anyone; it had the feeling of a new – or recovered – freedom. When I shut the door behind me, I felt as though I had forgotten something. Outside, my body seemed weightless in the sunshine, as though my feet were barely touching the ground. An unfamiliar peace had settled upon the house – there were no more visitors and our days were undisturbed – yet it did not feel empty, although we were on our own for the first time in five months.

Stan needed to have the certificate of death. I walked to the surgery, embalmed in sunshine, to collect it. As she handed me the envelope, the receptionist gave me a look of sympathy and understanding. The expressionless finality of the document caught me unawares. I had been in a calm, existential limbo and was unprepared for the shock waves that it sent through me.

Rory: Three days on, I sat in front of a television camera at Sky talking about *Magic Kingdom*. I did eight down-the-line radio interviews and three bookshop signings in London. The next day I flew to Manchester, then Edinburgh. *En route* to a reading, my car was caught in a thunderstorm. All around me dazzling rainbows appeared, curving between the near and far lanes of the motorway, arching across the sky, and I felt that you were with me. When Katrin tried to call the hotel room that evening, the line was engaged.

'He's telling Joan about his day,' she thought.

Over the next weeks I concentrated on the publicity campaign, finished sieving through your papers, tried not to consider why the freezer was so full of ice cream. I glanced up at our bedroom window while cutting the grass, hoping to see your silhouette. I pulled down the blind in your room at night so the morning light wouldn't wake you. I felt as if you had simply flown away to Canada or Malaysia.

Then one month on, while driving home from a party, Katrin said, 'I don't feel Joan in the house any more.' About the same time a friend awoke to see a form – indistinct, light and calm – floating above her bed. 'That'll be Joan saying goodbye,' she said to herself.

Seven years. Seven years. Seven years on I remember so many details: our dreams and lunches, the weight of the Cottage keys in my pocket, maroon-haired Florence's inane chat, the pearls of dew glistening on winter hedges. Yet despite the intensity of my memories, I cannot see your face. I cannot hear your voice. I cannot picture your eyes. I find that the harder I try to evoke you, the further you recede from my senses. Perhaps there is a bridge to another world but – as far as I can see – it is nowhere to be found. If anything, the hereafter is a place of non-being, of nothing. Here in the real world I transcribe diaries, reconstruct conversations, stare at fading photographs, and come to understand my – and perhaps our – need for books. With your death, a richness, joy and complexity vanished, along with a consoling fantasy and my youth. In these pages I hold on to the clear wonder of our one-and-only lives, trying to give meaning to the common-place, defy the void and face the dark infinity inside our hearts.

Of course, neither God nor the elegies of John Donne can bring you back. William Penn's assertion that 'they that love beyond the world cannot be separated from it' will never be proved. Not one of your favourite authors or novels, not Frayn, Mahfouz or Shields, and especially not my *Magic Kingdom*, can restore what is forever lost. I believe only that you are gone and that we will never meet again. The other actors in our final drama remain vivid to me, but you – so long the central player in my life – are a ghost.

Katrin: This morning I watched the shadows of the house martins rush across your bed. Sitting at my desk where your armchair once stood, I listened to the sparrows chirping and squabbling in the Virginia creeper. You'd hardly recognize the garden today. The silver birches and sorbus have doubled in height. The clematis and the climbing rose have buried the pine beneath clumps of vigorous growth. Your geraniums and lupins, transplanted from the Cottage, are blooming. Nestled among the trees at the bottom of the garden, there's a playhouse.

Seven years ago, Rory fell into a chasm of uncertainty. Your simple funeral service brought the family together again in a last ritual of farewell. We gathered bouquets of flowers from our garden to adorn your coffin. We drove to Esher, your warm ashes at my feet, to your mother's grave. I used my hands, not the urn, to scatter you, to feel you one last time, to show my love.

Throughout your life Rory had nurtured a belief in the soul's immortality, in living on. He searched for clues, but without proof his frail fiction collapsed, shaking his core, turning him inwards, silencing him. All decisions seemed pointless. What difference would it make if we left for London at 9 or at 3? If we drove or took the train? If we returned together or separately? The closeness that had come from caring for you ended abruptly with this shared experience; the crushing grief he felt at losing you separated him from me, irretrievably I thought. While I knew his pain, I did not feel it myself; he was engulfed by a force as amorphous and inexplicable as the concept of infinity. I grieved for Rory, for his loss – of you, of certainty – for my own loss of him. There were no words by which I could reach him; a part of his own spirit had vanished with you.

Slowly Rory progressed through the stages of mourning. Denial and anger – even bargaining – preceded your death; acceptance finally emerged from a long tunnel of depression. But none of us could have foreseen how, at the moment of your death, as the birds swooped up beneath the eaves, he too wanted to fly; perhaps to go with you, perhaps to rise above the darkness of grief.

I was shocked by Rory's mad idea – which grew from that moment – to build and fly an aeroplane, and amazed by the daring of his creativity. Although I was horrified by the possible outcome, I had to believe that his instinct was right. Intuitively, I understood his need to ritualize his grief, to give it shape – and that my support was essential. If he could not be dissuaded (and believe me, I did try), I somehow had to ensure that he did it as safely as possible. I became an unwilling accomplice in its creation, unable really to communicate with Rory in his withdrawn state and unwilling to voice my own unequivocal feelings to anxious friends, who must have wondered at my apparent calm. In a bid to hold myself together, I talked about the idea in a matter-of-fact way, belying my true feelings, divorcing myself from its possibilities and from Rory's careless attitude to life. As we packed our car with tools and materials for the long journey south to Crete, the island where man first flew, I stamped on my fears and put aside my misgivings.

Six months later, through the heat, far down the runway, the fragile white aircraft we had made buzzed towards me at full throttle, preparing to take off. It is a moment that will stay with me forever. All my senses were focused on

Rory, a small figure in the open cockpit. As the wheels peeled off the hot tarmac, elation and fear flooded me. The aeroplane made a symbolic hop before nose-diving on to the runway with a splintering crunch. At the second of impact I was already running, heart in mouth, flip-flops slapping the hot tarmac, the Cretans' jokes about widow's weeds and insurance policies playing through my head. Finally, Rory's crazy laughter reached me, signalling an end to this chapter of the story.

Rory turned this experience into *Falling for Icarus* and has since written other books. In our Dorset garden we planted new lavenders, potentillas and a thriving herb garden. A pair of magpies nested in the pine, driving a pair of blackbirds from their home until Rory dismantled their nest. I left Fired Earth and put aside basketry to start teaching English. Roger Federer became the world No. 1 tennis player (Henman never won Wimbledon). Lewis Hamilton and Fernando Alonso are the F1 drivers to watch now. And we were finally blessed with a son – your grandson.

Next week it will be his fifth birthday. As he grows, boldly advancing through life, our focus has naturally shifted to his future, to looking forwards instead of backwards over our shoulders. The flinty pain of grief has been smoothed by the years, the poignant memories of your dying now a part of our lives and our family's history. Time has a meaning and function again; where it slowed and stopped when you died, it is now moving – now racing – inexorably forwards, carrying us all along until we too tip beyond the horizon. And words, so helpless against the inexpressibility of loss, have recovered their power to articulate, to resonate and to connect us to each other.

Often I picture your face framed by our bedroom window, watching the birds at the feeder below. From this favourite perch you observed the world you loved, shared in its richness, were reassured by its continuity. Now Rory and I stand here, watching Finn blowing bubbles in the garden, chasing them with Tess until they float above his head, beyond reach. We laugh together in delight, for Finn's spirit and energy, for this gift of time together.

The bubbles rise above us, defying gravity, as we watch them drift and climb above the roof, bursting or escaping into the ether. I think of you now, light and free as Finn's bubbles, as bright motes adrift on the winds in the sunshine, as birds on the wing, endlessly circling – as the turf and loam beneath my son's feet, a part of nature, perpetual and ever-changing.